# THE HEART FACTS
## What You Can Do to Keep a Healthy Heart

Norman K. Hollenberg, M.D., Ph.D.
with Ilana B. Hollenberg

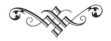

An AARP Book
published by
American Association of Retired Persons, Washington, D.C.
Scott, Foresman and Company, Glenview, Illinois

Copyright © 1989
Scott, Foresman and Company, Glenview, Illinois
American Association of Retired Persons, Washington, D.C.
All Rights Reserved
Printed in the United States of America

**Library of Congress Cataloging-in-Publication Data**

Hollenberg, Norman K.
    The heart facts / Norman K. Hollenberg with Ilana B. Hollenberg.
        p.    cm.
    Includes index.
    ISBN 0-673-24888-7
    1. Heart—Diseases—Popular works.    I. Hollenberg, Ilana B., 1962–
II. Title.
    RC681.H74  1988                                          88-14453
    616.1'2—dc19                                                 CIP

1 2 3 4 5 6-RRC-93 92 91 90 89 88

**AARP Books** provides interesting, timely, and practical information that enables persons 50 and over to improve the quality of their lives in their health, housing, finances, recreation, personal relationships, and work environment. These books are copublished by AARP, the world's largest membership and service organization for people 50 and over, and Scott, Foresman and Company, one of the nation's foremost educational publishers. For further information, contact AARP Books, 1900 East Lake Avenue, Glenview, IL 60025.

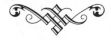

# Contents

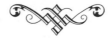

# Acknowledgments

Acknowledging the contributions of a series of individuals to the preparation of this manuscript is a very real pleasure. Without the persistent and persuasive efforts of Mr. Gerald Diamond, formerly of Biomedical Information Services, the project never would have been undertaken. Without the patient and skilled efforts of Ms. Diana Page and Mrs. Marie Bifolck, our notes would never have become a manuscript. Without the equally patient and skilled efforts of Mrs. Elaine Goldberg of Scott, Foresman and Company, the manuscript would not have become a book. We are grateful to Ms. Janice Swaine for her help with the preparation of tables on nutrition. The only difficult acknowledgment involves the many friends and colleagues who made helpful suggestions on the substance of the book, especially in areas of controversy and those demanding judgment. Here, there are too many to thank individually, and since none had an opportunity to review the manuscript, any remaining errors of judgment or fact can be attributed only to the authors. Finally, we are grateful to the following individuals, associations, companies, and publishers who granted us permission to use material for this text.

**Page 101** "Framingham Study Shows How Added Factors Multiply Risk" from "Heart Disease: Big Study Produces New Data" by Jane E. Brody, *The New York Times,* January 8, 1985, page C1. Copyright © 1985 by The New York Times Company. Reprinted by permission.

**Pages 101–102, 104–105** Quotations by Dr. Jeremiah Stamler from "Current Status of Dietary Prevention and Treatment of Atherosclerotic Coronary Artery Disease, *Progress in Cardiovascular Diseases* 3(1): 56–95, 1960.

**Page 102** "Cholesterol Ratio Is Clue to Heart Disease" from "Heart Disease: Big Study Produces New Data" by Jane E. Brody, *The New York Times,* January 8, 1985, page C1. Copyright © 1985 by The New York Times Company. Reprinted by permission.

**Page 103**   "Interrelationship Between Risk Factors and Cardiovascular Disease" from *The Nutrition Desk Reference* by Robert H. Garrison, Jr., M.A., R.Ph., and Elizabeth Somer, M.A., p. 151. Copyright © 1985 by Robert H. Garrison, Jr., and Elizabeth Somer. Reprinted by permission of Keats Publishing, Inc.

**Page 104**   "Combination of Risk Factors That Increases Danger of Heart Disease" adapted from *Your Healthy Heart* by Dr. Christiaan Barnard and Peter Evans. Copyright © 1985 by Multimedia Productions {UK} Ltd. Reprinted by permission.

**Page 117**   "Fatty Acid Composition of Oils and Fats" from *The Nutrition Desk Reference* by Robert H. Garrison, Jr., M.A., R.Ph., and Elizabeth Somer, M.A., p. 197. Copyright © 1985 by Robert H. Garrison, Jr., and Elizabeth Somer. Reprinted by permission of Keats Publishing, Inc.

**Page 120**   "Relationship of Serum Cholesterol to the Coronary Death Rate" from *The Nutrition Desk Reference* by Robert H. Garrison, Jr., M.A., R.Ph., and Elizabeth Somer, M.A., p. 160. Copyright © 1985 by Robert H. Garrison, Jr., and Elizabeth Somer. Reprinted by permission of Keats Publishing, Inc.

**Page 121**   "Cholesterol Content of Foods" from *The Nutrition Desk Reference* by Robert H. Garrison, Jr., M.A., R.Ph., and Elizabeth Somer, M.A., p. 198. Copyright © 1985 by Robert H. Garrison, Jr., and Elizabeth Somer. Reprinted by permission of Keats Publishing, Inc.

**Pages 122–123**   "Percentage of Fat Calories in Selected Foods" from *The Nutrition Desk Reference* by Robert H. Garrison, Jr., M.A., R.Ph., and Elizabeth Somer, M.A., pp. 201–202. Copyright © 1985 by Robert H. Garrison, Jr., and Elizabeth Somer. Reprinted by permission of Keats Publishing, Inc.

**Pages 126–127**   Height/Weight table adapted from *Statistical Bulletin*, Metropolitan Life Insurance Company, and information from the Gerontology Research Center of the National Institute on Aging. Reprinted by permission.

**Page 130**   "Calculate Your Target Heart Rate During Exercise." Adaptation of chart and text, "Target Heart Rate Calculator" by E. C. Frederick, Ph.D., and Stephen Kiesling, *American Health*, April, 1987, p. 36. Copyright © 1987 by American Health Partners. Reprinted by permission.

**Page 132**   "Cardiovascular Mortality" from *The Heart: The Living Pump* by Goode P. Davis, Jr., and Edwards Park and the Editors of U.S. News Books. Reprinted by permission of Marshall Editions.

**Page 164**   Adaptation of "Examples of ECG Readings" from *Your Healthy Heart* by Christiaan Barnard and Peter Evans. Copyright © 1985 by Multimedia Productions {UK} Ltd. Reprinted by permission.

**Page 177**   "Cutting Down on Sodium." Reproduced with permission. © *Cooking Without Your Salt Shaker*, American Heart Association.

**Pages 178–179**   "Sodium Content of Foods" from *The Nutrition Desk Reference* by Robert H. Garrison, Jr., M.A., R.Ph., and Elizabeth Somer, M.A., pp. 203–204. Copyright © 1985 by Robert H. Garrison, Jr., and Elizabeth Somer. Reprinted by permission of Keats Publishing, Inc.

**Page 239**   "Exercise and the Heart" from *The Heart: The Living Pump* by Goode P. Davis, Jr., and Edwards Park and the Editors of U.S. News Books. Reprinted by permission of Marshall Editions.

**Page 240**   "Popular Sports Among Americans Over 50" from "Here's how they stay in shape" in Parade Magazine, *Boston Globe*, December 1, 1985. Reprinted by permission of Lloyd Shearer.

**Page 242**   "If You're Not Ready to Quit—Tips from the Addiction Research Foundation" from *Tar and Nicotine Ratings May Be Hazardous to Your Health: Information for Smokers Who Are Not Ready to Stop" by Lynn T. Kozlowski, Ph.D. Copyright © 1982 Alcohol and Drug Addiction Research Foundation, Toronto, Canada. Reprinted by permission.

**Pages 261–264**   "What Kinds of Services Are Available?" and "How to Choose a Home Care Agency." Adaptations from brochure *How to Choose a Home Care Agency: A Consumer's Guide and Patient's Bill of Rights.* Reprinted by permission of the National Association for Home Care.

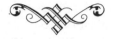

# Preface

Diseases of the heart and the circulatory system are widely recognized as the leading cause of death and disability in the United States today. Cardiovascular diseases kill twice as many people each year as cancer and ten times as many as accidents. The largest number, 55 percent, die of heart attacks—followed by strokes, high blood pressure, and rheumatic fever. One-fifth of the people who succumb to cardiovascular disease are under the age of sixty-five.

High blood pressure is a problem for nearly 58 million people in the United States, and more than 63 million Americans—or one in four people—suffer from some form of cardiovascular disease. The figure is one in two for people over age sixty-five. Coronary artery disease is common. An estimated 191,000 coronary bypass operations were performed in 1983, and the number is expected to increase to 400,000 in 1995. Despite that extraordinary number, only a fraction of those suffering from coronary artery disease will come to surgery.

At a recent symposium, it was estimated that we would add as much as eighteen years to the average American life span if we could stamp out diseases of the heart and the circulatory system, and only two or three years to the life span if we could stamp out cancer. This, too, reflects the fact that many relatively young people succumb to the impact of cardiovascular diseases.

What do we spend on cardiovascular disease? Reasonable estimates—perhaps conservative—indicate that over 80 billion dollars was spent in 1986 for diseases of the circulatory system, about $325 for every man, woman, and child in the United States. These are not approximate figures; the costs include 48.2 billion dollars for hospital and nursing home services, 13.6

billion dollars for lost work due to disability, 11.8 billion dollars for doctor bills, and 6 to 8 billion dollars for medications.

There is, however, substantial good news. The outlook has improved. Deaths from all forms of cardiovascular disease declined by 31 percent between 1972 and 1983. The decline has been attributed to such lifestyle changes as better diet, exercise, and reduced cigarette smoking even more than it has been to improved medical care. That is not to ignore the impact of improved medical care. The striking reduction in stroke, kidney failure, and heart failure due to hypertension is attributable largely to more effective therapy.

Much is preventable with what is known today. The major point of this book will be an attempt to extend and improve upon that 31 percent reduction by providing practical guidelines and tips for keeping your heart healthy.

The goal is to describe what is known, give some indication as to how confident researchers are with the information, provide some useful information on what you can do to prevent problems, and provide insight into what the physician is doing when he or she makes suggestions about diagnostic procedures, medical therapy, or surgery. Cost of drugs, their safety and dependability, and the likelihood of taking unneeded medication will also be addressed. Special emphasis will be given to material that is especially relevant to the individual fifty years of age or older.

# 1

# "Normal" Aging and Well-Being

According to the National Center for Health Statistics, every day about five thousand Americans celebrate their sixty-fifth birthdays. The nation has over 29 million senior citizens, most of them between the ages of fifty and sixty-five.

Dr. T. Franklin Williams, director of the National Institute on Aging, at Bethesda, Maryland, recently said, "The idea of the second fifty years is beginning to gain wide acceptance . . . the day is coming when middle age will begin to end on an individual's seventy-fifth birthday."

Some individuals age particularly well. Outstanding examples include Winston Churchill, Charles de Gaulle, Konrad Adenauer, Maggie Kuhn, Pablo Casals, Lillian Gish, and George Burns. Their vitality and energy allowed them to hold tough jobs and produce while in their eighties. Chronological age is not a reliable indicator of how a person will function.

An important study, the Baltimore Longitudinal Study on Aging, was initiated in 1958. In this study, the same individuals have been examined repeatedly over a prolonged period to allow researchers to learn what happens as people age. James L. Fozzard, Ph.D., associate science director of that program, has pointed out that "the general public has the mistaken idea that aging is a disease. Poor health is not an inevitable consequence of old age. Instead, aging is a lifelong process . . . the public can make daily decisions which will influence their health and vitality, more than all of today's medicines."

## WHAT IS "NORMAL"

Words such as *normal*, *abnormal*, *health*, and *disease* are employed so frequently that we intuitively believe that we understand them. Words used by different people, however, may carry different meanings. For example, many will remember the acronym SNAFU, widely used by members of the armed services in World War II. The letters meant "Situation Normal, All Fouled Up." In other words, in a large and hastily organized bureaucracy, the normal situation was chaos.

What about the application of the word *normal* to the question of well-being? Several hundred years ago the average life span was eighteen years; eighteen was the "normal" age to die. In ancient Rome, the wealthy could afford the best. The best included piped-in water and high-quality wine. The origin of our word *plumbing* is the Latin word for lead—the first metal that could be worked as pipes. Lead containers were also used to store the best wine, and lead was used to sweeten and preserve the wine. Thus, the more wealthy one was, the more likely it was that one suffered the long-term consequences of prolonged lead exposure. Chronic lead poisoning was so prevalent among the leading citizens at that time that some have suggested that the fall of the Roman Empire really reflected destruction of its leadership by wealth-engendered lead poisoning! It was so common that the disease state could be considered "normal." An older adult male of a wealthy family who did not have lead poisoning was considered "abnormal."

A dictionary definition of health generally involves being "sound in body, mind, and spirit," with special emphasis on freedom from physical disease. Disease is a physical or mental derangement, reflecting a degree of impaired performance of a vital function.

### Aging and the "Normal"

These definitions are all well and good, but they raise a problem. How much deviation from well-being is required for health to become disease? Equally important, how much should doctors adjust their decisions according to how old a patient is? Doctors spend too much time saying that some item is appropriate to an individual's age, and thus dismissing it.

### Probability and the "Normal Range"

For scientists and physicians, the word *probability* has only one meaning—how often something will happen. An event that occurs one time in a million is obviously rare. If an event occurs one time in three, that is obviously common. Somewhere between a very common event (typical) and a very rare event (atypical) is a dividing line. Somewhat arbitrarily, the decision has been made that one time in twenty will be considered the standard dividing atypical from typical. Obviously, if an event occurs one time in a hundred, or one time in a thousand, we can be more confident that the observation is atypical.

These concepts are used in evaluating the results of all tests used by physicians. In each case a "normal range"—that is, the range of test results that will be considered normal—is established.

## TESTING FOR THE "NORMAL RANGE"

How is the normal range determined in medicine? Let us examine what happened when someone found a way to measure blood sugar concentration with a chemical test for the first time. Doctors already knew that patients with diabetes mellitus (which means the person produces a large volume of sweet urine) had a substantial amount of sugar (glucose) in their urine. They quickly discovered with their new blood test that most individuals with a great deal of glucose in their urine also had a very high concentration of glucose in their blood. This, indeed, is how they learned that the cause of glucose in the urine is a high concentration of glucose in the blood. They also found that most individuals who do not have sugar in their urine have a much lower blood sugar level. The "normal range" of blood sugar was identified as the blood sugar found in 95 percent of the population, the common value for all tests.

What of the individuals who did not have sugar in their urine but whose blood sugar seemed somewhat high? Well, when the test was first developed, it was unclear where their trouble lay. With time, after measuring their blood sugar repeatedly, follow-up studies showed what happened to them. Many went on to have the well-known characteristics of diabetes, including sugar in the urine. Thus, the ability to make

---

Chronological age is not a reliable indicator of how a person will function.

the measurement at first raised some troubling problems but later extended insight into the disease.

## The Screening Test and False Positives

The concept of the normal range raises a number of questions. If a laboratory does the test twenty times, once in twenty times—by chance—the result will lie outside the "normal" range. Similarly, if one performs twenty tests on an individual, by chance one of them may lie outside that range. The likelihood that the test really reflects a disease involves a number of factors including *how* abnormal the test result is and what other information is available that suggests that the result really does reflect an abnormality. For example, if one has a history of exposure to someone with hepatitis, an abnormal result in one of the liver function tests is more likely to reflect an abnormality in the liver. If more than one test of liver function is abnormal, the likelihood that each truly reflects a liver disease also increases.

This concept has especially important implications for what have come to be called "screening" tests. These are tests that are performed in an apparently healthy individual, without symptoms, to detect early disease. There are real problems with this approach, based on the statistical considerations discussed above.

Let us take as an example a simple test for a disease that is reasonably common, that is, that occurs in the community with a frequency of about 1 in 1,000 individuals. Because the normal range reflects the results in 19 of 20 apparently healthy individuals, there will be a "false positive rate" of 5 percent. In other words, 5 percent of the time the test will appear to be positive though the individual is healthy.

Let us take an apparently healthy individual, perform the test, and find a positive result. What is the likelihood that the

---

**DEFINING THE "ATYPICAL"**

Somewhat arbitrarily, the decision has been made that one time in twenty will be considered the minimum criterion for dividing the atypical from the typical. An event that occurs only one time in twenty is thus atypical. This concept is used in all the tests employed by doctors—it is the basis for the "normal range."

**FALSE POSITIVES**

If scientists perform a test 1,000 times, the 5 percent false positive rate means that they would find 50 positive tests. If the disease occurs in 1 in 1,000, only 1 of those 50 will prove to actually have the disease.

individual, in fact, has the disease? The probability of the individual actually having the disease is only 2 percent. How do we come to that conclusion? If we perform the test 1,000 times, the 5 percent false positive rate means that we would find 50 positive tests. However, the disease has only a frequency of 1 in a 1,000, so only 1 of the 50 would actually have the disease.

Obviously, a probability of 2 percent, that is 2 in 100, is higher than the probability of 1 in 1,000 that we began with, but it is still unlikely that the positive test, in fact, reflects disease.

This is such a common sequence that virtually anyone who sees a physician regularly has had the experience. What can the physician do? The first thing that the physician may do is repeat the test. If the result of the test is due to random fluctuation, the next test will generally be in the normal range. Often another kind of test will also be performed. If, in fact, a disease is present, the second test will also show an abnormality. Particularly if the test is borderline abnormal, the prudent physician will often suggest that it be repeated in three months.

## The Logic of Routine Screening

These concepts underlie some of the controversy that you may have read about regarding the usefulness of routine screening. On the one hand, it is obviously better to identify high blood pressure and diabetes before they have done their damage. If we can find a cancer before it has spread, and many cancers can be found early during a physical examination, we have obviously accomplished a great deal. In the past, hyperparathyroidism, a disease of the parathyroid glands, was remembered by medical students as "bones and stones." When diagnosis of hyperparathyroidism was made, the patient already had advanced bone disease or evidence of kidney stones. Today, because serum calcium and serum phosphorous are measured as part of health examinations, the disease is most often identified early, when the patient begins to show an increase in serum calcium but before the damage to the bones and the kidneys occurs. All of these things are a plus.

For every positive finding and test that turns out to be a clue to early disease—and a therapeutic triumph—doctors find many tests that are false and that lead to worry and expense. This is not a fault of the tests; rather, it is built into the logic of the system. All doctors can do is be patient as they sort out the various possible meanings of a positive test result.

Let us take a common example. The life insurance examination often turns up something, but more often than not the initial observation is incorrect. For that reason, the insurance company will often play the "statistics game" and, especially for younger individuals, enlist them without much evaluation. The cost of chasing down each test result turns out to be greater than the cost of insuring the occasional individual who should not have been insured.

## ADJUSTMENT FOR AGE?

In evaluating test results, how much, if at all, should we adjust for the age of the person being tested? At one end of the age spectrum—infants and children, for example—it is obviously critical to judge important characteristics as a function of age. A child developing normally should be able to hold its head up at a certain stage, follow with its eyes at a certain stage, begin to crawl and walk at certain stages, and begin to use language at a certain stage. Every parent, and every pediatrician, follows these developments with great excitement.

When dealing with older persons, however, it is by no means clear that adjustment for age is routinely a useful approach. Accepting the fact that lead-related symptoms occurred with increasing age was obviously not in the Roman's best interest. It was far better to identify the lead problem and deal with it. A host of conditions occur with sufficient frequency in an aging population that adjustment for age has become commonplace. In Western society, blood pressure tends to rise with age. Is an elevated blood pressure normal? Weight tends to increase with age. Is overweight necessary? The bones tend to become thinner with age and prone to fracture. Is osteoporosis a necessary accompaniment of age?

Just as it was not a good idea for the Romans to consider the symptoms of lead poisoning normal with increasing age, it is a mistake to consider an elevated blood pressure normal in an older individual.

The answer in each case is no. Let us take the question of blood pressure as an example. In every study performed in a highly structured society—that is, a society that has given rise to cities—the average blood pressure in the community increases with age. By the same token, the number of individuals in whom the blood pressure can be considered high—that is, above the normal range—increases. The observation of high blood pressure is so common that many formulas were constructed to identify what should be considered high blood pressure in older individuals.

Just as it was not a good idea to consider the symptoms of lead poisoning normal with increasing age, it is no wiser to consider an elevated blood pressure healthy in an older individual just because it is common. First, studies have shown that for individuals who live in a less cluttered society, away from cities, and who typically eat a restricted salt diet, blood pressure does not increase with age. When individuals from such cultures move into an urban society, they "catch" high blood pressure with increasing age.

Second, the results of another study show that high blood pressure in older persons can and should be treated. The final link in the evidence comes from recent studies on the treatment of high blood pressure in the elderly. In mid-1985, the widely read British medical journal *The Lancet* published a study from the European Working Party Trial on Hypertension in the Elderly (see page 8). A large number of individuals with hypertension were either treated with drugs or a placebo (an innocuous substance) for an average of seven years. The question was, Did treatment reduce the likelihood of hypertension-related effects? The answer was a clear yes. Despite the fact that the individuals treated were in their seventies, the likelihood of their having a stroke or of dying from a heart attack was reduced sharply with treatment. Although blood pressure might typically increase with age, that is not to be considered normal or healthy. Elevation in blood pressure merits treatment.

Similar arguments apply to the question of increasing body weight with age, to the question of loss of bone mass in the elderly woman, and to virtually every other condition commonly associated with age. The task of the medical profession is to see what can be done to prevent the problem, wherever possible, and what the best approach to treatment is when prevention is impossible.

Another important study took place in Alameda County, California. It lasted ten years and included a scientific sampling of seven thousand men and women. They showed that by observing a few positive health practices, a forty-five-year-old man could expect to live eleven years longer, and a forty-five-year-old woman seven years longer, than a person who did not make those same choices. Not only could they live longer, but it is also likely that they could *enjoy* those years more. The recommended health practices in the study were commonplace: the individual had to get enough sleep, get enough exercise, give up cigarettes, consume alcohol only in moderation, maintain a proper weight, and eat a hearty breakfast. This may not be new advice, but it apparently still holds true.

## AGING AND TREATMENT OF DISEASE

Broad advances are being made in both the prevention and the treatment of health-related problems in the older individual. Some changes do occur in the body when we have used it for many years, and these changes have implications when prescribing appropriate treatment. Fortunately, there has been increasing interest in the study of how and whether the aging process influences treatment for common conditions.

An outstanding contemporary example is the recent report just cited from the European Working Party Trial on Hypertension in the Elderly, a group based in Europe, on treatment of high blood pressure in the individual who is sixty years of age or older. This was an ambitious study, opened in 1972 and not completed until 1984. The study questioned how effective treatment for high blood pressure was when instituted in the individual who is over sixty years of age. The question was not just, Could blood pressure be lowered? Scientists knew the answer to that. The question was, Did reduction of blood pressure influence the natural course of the condition the way it did in younger individuals? Could one prevent strokes? Could treatment reduce the likelihood of having a heart attack? If one had a heart attack, could treatment reduce the risk that one would die from it? Could treatment prevent congestive heart failure?

The answers provided by this study can be seen as good news. The drugs were as well tolerated by older individuals as they are by younger. The likelihood that the treated individual would suffer a stroke or die from a heart attack was reduced sharply.

**Drugs in Older Persons**

With increasing age, a number of changes occur that can have implications for the use of drugs. One important change involves kidney function. There is a small but clear reduction in kidney function that becomes apparent when an individual reaches his or her forties. Thereafter, about 10 percent of kidney function is lost for every ten years of age. Since many drugs are eliminated by the kidney, the result is that for many drugs it is appropriate to adjust the dose downward.

There may also be an increased sensitivity to the action of a drug, even if its elimination is not altered. One example is the influence of drugs that reduce blood pressure. Many persons show, normally, a small fall in blood pressure when they move from the sitting or recumbent to the standing position. In older persons, blood pressure fall tends to be greater, especially the first thing in the morning or after a heavy meal. If to that fall in blood pressure that occurs with standing, one adds a blood pressure fall due to a drug or to alcohol, the result may be a much larger fall in blood pressure and a feeling of dizziness.

## QUALITY OF LIFE

Treatability of a condition is not the only concern of health care consumers and providers, however. Quality of life has emerged as a prominent concern in the field of health care due in part to the enormous increase in the relative proportion of chronic conditions such as heart disease, hypertension, arthritis, and diabetes as our population grows older. For these conditions, the chances of cure are small, and longevity is often not the most appropriate indicator of effectiveness of health measures. The use of medications for treatment of these conditions may extend life, or may not, but what price should one pay to make life longer with a drug that causes depression and so diminishes the quality of life?

We tend to think of drug side effects in terms of a rash,

nausea, or constipation — or a host of such things. Too little attention has been paid to how medications affect the person's feelings of well-being, mood, and sexual function. The patient too rarely mentions these side effects to the physician; the physician too rarely asks about them.

As one example, it is not enough for a drug to reduce blood pressure today; it must achieve this goal without sacrificing the individual's function socially, emotionally, and intellectually.

In the search for cure, treatment, and quality of life, expectations must be tempered with reality, of course, and caution must be a byword.

## CAUTION WITH NEW CONCEPTS

We live in a high-technology culture but still carry around an enormous number of primitive beliefs. Since the time of Andrew Jackson, Americans have been as likely to respond to self-proclaimed messiahs of health as they are to the best available advice based on solid information. An enormous amount of time and expense has been invested in a host of silly miracle cures.

Gullibility, as seen in the current purchase of books supporting one fad or another, has long been evident. Snake oil was the common cure-all for years. Less than a century ago, Horace Fletcher claimed that obesity and leanness, indigestion and bleeding piles, and even skin eruptions could be cured by chewing one's food until it was a tasteless pulp. Eating bean sprouts had its day. A recent version involves chelation for the treatment of atherosclerosis. Physicians use a number of drugs that chelate (that is, bind) to heavy metal for a number of purposes in medicine, but especially for the removal of heavy metals, such as lead, aluminum, and copper. In the patient with Wilson's disease, for example, there is an abnormality in copper metabolism that makes chelates very attractive for removal of the copper. A similar logic can apply to lead poisoning. Presumably, because of the calcium seen under the microscope in atherosclerotic arteries, it has been suggested that the drugs used for chelating might be useful for atherosclerosis. There is not a bit of evidence to indicate that these drugs reverse atherosclerosis, and there is clear evidence that they can be toxic. Despite the absence of evidence, information continues to appear in the lay press promoting this new form of quackery.

Physicians are not immune to fads. Once they recom-

mended the removal of all of the teeth, the removal of the colon, or suspension of the uterus. Before you sneer, do you know
someone with arthritis who currently wears a copper brace-
let? How are we to know which messiah provides us with solid
information?

For example, the claim that eating fish can prevent heart
attacks is not a new one but has received much recent attention. Why should we believe that eating cold water fish, fish oil,
or fifteen capsules of eicosapentaenoic acid (EPA) every day will
improve our health? How does fish oil differ from snake oil?

The first clue to the value of fish in preventing heart attacks
goes back to an observation made over thirty years ago. Eskimos living in Greenland were found to have a very low frequency of heart attack and of hardening of the arteries despite
the fact that they consumed a high-calorie, high-fat diet. One
of the ways they differ from their southern neighbors is in what
they eat. But, that, of course, is not the only difference. Their
work patterns, sleep patterns, social interactions, and climate
also differ. To avoid heart attacks, should we all move to the
Arctic Circle? The observation on heart attacks in the Eskimo
provided a clue suggesting where we ought to look but no clear
indication as to what lifestyle change we ought to make. Indeed,
it was possible that the difference was genetic, built into Eskimo genes, and impossible to mimic with any lifestyle change.

Several lines of investigation were undertaken to examine
the possibility that fish in the diet played a role. One line of
investigation involved an exploration of the fatty components
in fish, in comparison with the fatty components in meat. These
investigations revealed that the fatty acids in fish differ substantially from the fatty acids in meat. Then it was found that
replacing the dietary fatty acids obtained from meat with fatty
acids from fish, such as eicosapentaenoic acid, changed the
function and composition of platelets and fats in the bloodstream of people. Did this prove that doing so is useful? By no
means. These maneuvers merely were the first step in developing the evidence that changing one's diet could change the body,

"The idea of the second fifty years is beginning to gain wide acceptance . . .
the day is coming when middle age will begin to end on an individual's
seventy-fifth birthday."

—Dr. T. Franklin Williams

---

**PREVENTABLE CARDIOVASCULAR DISORDERS**

- Heart attack
- Stroke
- High blood pressure
- Rheumatic fever

---

and in a direction that could be useful. There were more steps to follow. Epidemiological research was necessary to trace the background of heart attacks. Studies had to be undertaken — either cross-sectional or longitudinal. The findings of large numbers of individuals regarding frequency of disease and factors that might influence it had to be examined.

## Cross-sectional Studies

In one form of epidemiological research, cross-sectional, a large number of individuals who have a problem, such as coronary heart disease, are matched with a large number of individuals who appear not to have that problem but who are the same age, sex, and social class and who have as many like characteristics as can be matched.

If a difference between the groups is found, such as the amount of fish that is eaten, maybe the fish is responsible for the difference. To make the assessment more powerful, one can examine the frequency of other factors thought to contribute to risk, such as overweight, family history of heart disease, cigarette smoking, hypertension, and high blood cholesterol. The weakness of this approach obviously involves the limited nature of that list. Can we statistically correct for all the possible risk factors? Clearly, we cannot, so information from cross-sectional studies is limited. A much more powerful technique is longitudinal study.

## Longitudinal Studies

A longitudinal study compares groups of individuals over a long period of time. Ideally, people are randomly assigned to two or more groups so that they are much more likely to be similar in every way, except for the one factor that is made different. Since this technique is so much better, why would anyone do a cross-sectional study? If an individual has an idea to be tested, a cross-sectional study can be organized in a relatively short time; a large number of individuals can be examined; and an answer can be provided within a short time, perhaps a couple of years. If a longitudinal study requires fifteen to twenty years, the answer cannot become available for a long time. A longitudinal study is much more expensive to set up and is sensitive to the possibility participants will drop out of the study—providing a much weaker answer. In general, longitudinal studies are much less common and are rarely undertaken until cross-sectional studies provide a strong indication that they should be.

Now, back to the fish story. The cross-sectional studies on fish intake led to a very important longitudinal investigation in Holland, in the Zutphen area. Here, individuals were enrolled in the early 1960s for a study on their mortality; the results of that study were published in the *New England Journal of Medicine* in May, 1985. This longitudinal study provided strong evidence that individuals who ate fish regularly had a striking reduction in the frequency of death from heart attack. Even more striking was the relation between the amount of fish that had been eaten and the likelihood of a fatal heart attack. There seemed to be little gain from eating more than 450 grams of fish a week—about two typical fish dinners—though eating much less than that clearly exerted less benefit. The good news was not only that eating fish was effective but that one need not consume an enormous amount of fish.

Is the evidence absolutely foolproof? No. To nail the evidence down, we would need the results of one more study. In that study, individuals at risk of coronary heart disease would be assigned, randomly, to treatments that included fish or excluded it. We would follow these two groups of individuals for the ten or twenty years required to accumulate a sufficient experience in heart attacks and determine whether the two groups showed a different frequency.

---

**GOOD NEWS**

Deaths from all forms of cardiovascular disease declined by 31 percent between 1972 and 1983. Better diet, more exercise, control of high blood pressure, and reduced cigarette smoking have made much of the difference.

---

Are we likely to do that study? No. How can we ensure that the groups assigned to not eating fish will agree to do so? How can we get individuals in a free society to participate in this kind of controlled study? Does that mean things are hopeless? No. It means that we have to recognize that the best available evidence is often imperfect. In this case, the evidence isn't bad.

## Making Practical Use of the Evidence

Does that mean that we should all be taking fifteen or more capsules of eicosapentaenoic acid every day? Certainly EPA is being marketed, and a large number of individuals are buying these capsules from health food stores. Still, the answer is no. There is no clear evidence that it was the eicosapentaenoic acid in fish that did the trick. Indeed, there are other candidates as the beneficial agent among the fish fatty acids, and it wouldn't at all be surprising if something other than fatty acids in fish contributed to well-being. The best solution, clearly, is to enjoy fish regularly. It didn't take that much fish in the Zutphen study to reduce risk.

# 2

# How the Cardiovascular System Works

Many medical historians believe that the influence of modern physiology on medical theory and practice began with William Harvey's first description of the circulation of the blood more than 300 years ago. Certainly our modern understanding of how the body works grew from that observation. Harvey's description was such an outstanding breakthrough in part because it came before the discovery of the microscope. The blood leaves the heart by way of the arteries and returns to the heart by way of the veins. The blood vessels that connect the arteries and veins, the tiny capillaries in every organ, are far too small to be seen with the naked eye. William Harvey guessed that they had to be present to complete the circulation; that guess was brilliant. They are not only present in every organ, but they also represent the essence of the circulation—the delivery of fresh blood to the capillaries and removal of waste products.

The capillaries represent the pathway for the delivery of oxygen and various nutrients to every cell in every organ in the body and the route by which waste substances are removed from the tissues. There are few tissues in the body where individual cells are more than one or two cell layers away from a capillary. Without capillaries, no organ could be more than about one millimeter in thickness, as that represents the limit for diffusion, or movement, of oxygen and the nutrients into the cell and for the diffusion of carbon dioxide and other waste products away from the cell.

## THE HEART AS A PUMP

Despite its importance, the heart is one of the simplest organs in the body. It has primarily a mechanical function—it serves as a pump. The heart is almost pure muscle. Every time the muscle contracts, it squeezes the blood in the heart, placing it under pressure and forcing it through the arteries to the capillaries. The pressure from the heart pushes the blood along, very much like squeezing a tube of toothpaste forces the toothpaste out.

The heart has four chambers. Blood returning to the veins from the various organs in the body has been depleted of oxygen and has had carbon dioxide, a waste product of body metabolism, added to it. The blood in the veins pours into the right side of the heart—first the right atrium and then the right ventricle. When the right ventricle contracts, as it does with each beat of the heart, it forces the blood through the arteries to

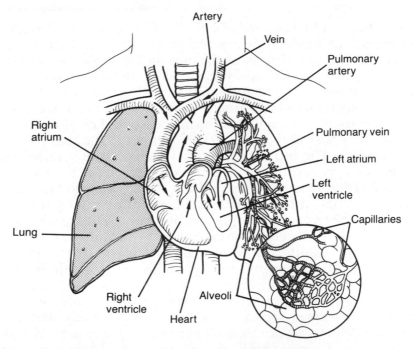

**Figure 1.   The Circulation Through the Heart and Lungs**

The blood coming from the veins flows through the right atrium, right ventricle, and pulmonary artery to the lung capillaries, where oxygen is taken up and carbon dioxide is removed. From there the blood flows back through the pulmonary veins to the left atrium and ventricle and then to the arteries of the body.

the lungs and into the lung capillaries. This is known as the pulmonary circulation (see figures 1 and 2). As the blood trickles through the capillaries in the lung, the carbon dioxide leaves to enter the lung air and be breathed out. Each breath blows away the carbon dioxide and brings fresh oxygen into the lungs; that oxygen enters the blood in the pulmonary capillaries, turning the blood bright red.

The blood then enters another two heart chambers—first the left atrium and then the left ventricle. When the left ventricle contracts (see figure 3), it squeezes blood into the large arteries, creating blood pressure. The blood is delivered by the arteries to every organ in the body, providing oxygen and nutrition and removing waste products. The specifics of blood pressure physiology are discussed in detail in chapter 5.

## THE LARGE ARTERIES

The blood forced out of the heart enters a system of branched, muscular tubes, the large arteries. The first large artery is the aorta, and all the arterial blood supply to every organ of the body originates from branches of the aorta. The first branches are the coronary arteries, the blood supply to the heart, closely

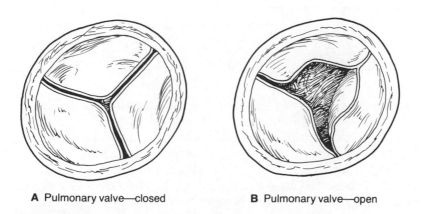

**A** Pulmonary valve—closed      **B** Pulmonary valve—open

**Figure 2.  Pulmonary Valve of the Heart**

The pulmonary valve separates the right ventricle from the pulmonary artery. Valve leaflets are closed **(A)**, preventing backward flow of blood from the pulmonary artery into the right ventricle. The right ventricle is contracting **(B)**, and blood is forced through the open valve into the pulmonary artery.

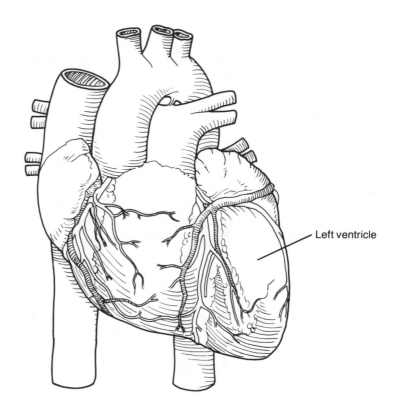

Left ventricle

**Figure 3.   Front of the Heart**
The left ventricle is in the front and is the part of the heart that one can feel as a thrust on the left side of the chest when the heart contracts.

followed by the arteries to the arms and the head. The aorta continues through the chest, giving off branches to the muscles, skin, and spinal cord, and when the abdomen is reached, further branches to the liver, stomach, intestines, spleen, and kidneys. Finally, the aorta terminates in the lower abdomen, dividing into two branches that go to the legs. The series of branchings and subbranchings resembles a tree, and the term *arterial tree* is widely used.

The function of the large arteries is to act as a series of conduits, carrying blood to all the organs, and to turn a discontinuous, or intermittent, flow of blood from the heart into the arteries to a continuous flow of blood from the arteries into the capillaries (see figure 4).

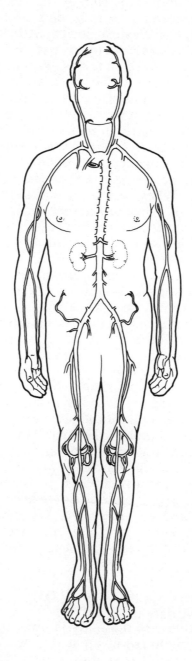

**Figure 4.   The Arterial System**

Despite the simple function of the arteries, disease of the large arteries represents the most common cause of death and disability in people of Western society. Atherosclerosis (detailed in chapter 7) occurs as a series of patches, called plaques, in large- and medium-sized arteries. When a large amount of atherosclerosis is present, the aorta and its branches become less flexible, and pressure rises. As atherosclerotic plaques become larger, they take up space within the artery, causing obstruction. By replacing the normal lining of the artery, which has as its major function the prevention of clot formation, atherosclerotic plaques lead to blood clots that block the artery and thereby destroy the tissue the artery normally supplied with blood. When that occurs in the blood supply to the heart, the result is coronary artery disease, angina pectoris, or myocardial infarction (see chapters 7, 9, and 10). When that occurs in the blood supply to the brain, the result is a stroke (see chapter 14). When the blood supply to the limb is involved in this way, the result is peripheral arterial disease and intermittent claudication (see chapter 15). When that occurs in the blood supply to the kidneys, the result is renal artery stenosis and renal vascular hypertension (see chapter 6). Less commonly, the blood supply to the intestines is involved with this process, and the result is mesenteric angina. Since the need for blood flow typically increases when an organ is exercising its function, it should not be surprising that the patient with mesenteric angina will tend to have pain in the abdomen after meals.

A substantial amount of the preventive measures examined in this book are related to the problem of atherosclerosis.

Less common, but an important problem involving the larger arteries is the formation of aneurysms (swellings). If a large artery develops a weakness, the pressure inside the artery tends to cause it to balloon out. This area of widening and weakness is called an aneurysm. When aneurysms become larger, there is the risk that they will burst, resulting in excessive bleeding and typically in a rapid death.

## BLOOD FLOW

The total blood flow to the body is obviously the same as the total output of blood from the heart—the cardiac output. Every organ or tissue has a certain minimal blood flow requirement when it is at rest and an increased requirement when it is performing work. Blood flow to the skeletal muscle or to the heart is substantially lower when one is resting, for example, than during active exercise. Clearly, if all of the body was to receive its maximal flow all of the time, the cardiovascular system would need a fundamentally different structure, capable of delivering much more blood flow.

The effect of eating a meal on blood flow to the intestines was mentioned earlier. Let us examine another situation. With exercise, the metabolic requirements of the exercising muscle increase dramatically. To fill that increase in metabolic need, the blood flow to the exercising muscle increases. At the same time, blood flow to other organs such as the kidney and intestines decreases. In that way, the increase in need is met in part by an increase in cardiac output and in part by redirecting or redistributing blood flow from one organ to another.

To take another example, exposure to heat results in a large increase in blood flow to the skin to help dissipate the body heat. Blood, as it leaves the heart, has the same temperature as the rest of the core of the body, about 97.6° Fahrenheit, and the temperature of the skin is far lower. When there is a need to dissipate heat, an increase of blood flow to the skin will result in increased delivery of heat, raising the local skin temperature and thus allowing the skin to radiate more heat. A similar phenomenon occurs during a fever. Again, blood flow elsewhere falls at the same time as blood flow to the skin increases.

When more blood flow is required by one organ, less is available to another. Everyone has been cautioned about swimming immediately after eating a heavy meal, since the likelihood of competition for blood flow will increase the probability of having serious muscle cramps. The less fit one is, the more of a problem that tends to be. A similar problem would accompany any form of exercise, including becoming sexually active, after a heavy meal.

## THE ARTERIOLES

The arteries become smaller and smaller through a series of progressive branching until they become very tiny immediately before they branch into capillaries. These small arteries are called arterioles (see figure 5). Relative to their size, they have a thick, smooth muscle coat and are capable of very strong contraction. The smallest arterioles represent the major factor determining where blood flow will be delivered. When the smooth

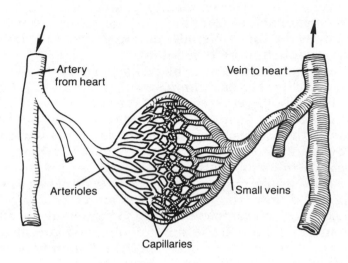

**Figure 5.    The Capillary Circulation**

Blood flows from the heart to the arteries and from there to small arteries called arterioles to the capillaries. Fresh blood in the capillaries supplies the body's cells with oxygen and nutrients and picks up for removal waste products and carbon dioxide. From the capillaries, the blood flows through small veins into larger veins and then to the heart, where the circulation begins again.

muscles in the walls of the arterioles to one organ contract, the result is an increased resistance to blood flow through the arterioles, and thus a decrease in the blood flow. On the other hand, if the blood arterioles to an organ relax, they increase the size of their bore, and will allow a larger blood flow. In this way, blood flow can be redirected from one site to another.

The arterioles are thus responsible for redirecting blood flow from one organ to another. The arterioles in the area requiring an increase in blood flow open up (dilate), and the arterioles in other parts of the body close down somewhat (constrict) and thus limit blood flow to those regions. If all the arterioles constrict without dilation in other organs, the result is an increase in arterial blood pressure—analogous to closing a dam so that the pressure and volume build up on the inflow side of the dam. The arterioles thus participate in the problem of hypertension.

## THE CAPILLARIES

The capillaries are very tiny tubes with a diameter very little larger than the diameter of a red blood cell. Because they are very thin-walled, they allow the rapid exchange of nutrients in the fresh inflowing arterial blood to the tissues, while material accumulated in the tissues diffuses to the blood in the capillaries. The result is that oxygen, sugar, fatty acids, hormones, vitamins, minerals, and other critical factors required by the tissues are delivered. At the same time, the blood leaving tissue has accumulated the waste products of metabolism, such as carbon dioxide and the breakdown products of fats and proteins, to be delivered to the lung, the kidney, and the liver for excretion.

There are few diseases of the capillaries. The swelling that occurs during inflammation, or with allergy, reflects the presence of temporarily "leaky" capillaries that enable the fluid and protein contained in the blood to run into the tissues.

## THE VEINS

As the blood leaves the capillaries, it enters a progressively larger series of tubes, the veins, that return the blood to the heart (see figure 6). Veins differ from arteries in several important ways. Once the blood has been through the arterioles and capillaries, the remaining blood pressure is very much lower. It is a general rule that the higher the blood pressure within a blood vessel, the thicker its wall will be. As a consequence, veins tend to be much more thin-walled. The blood they contain is no longer red, since a substantial amount of the oxygen has been removed in the capillaries. That is why the veins appear to be blue. The skin veins are often visible, especially in the backs of the hands, the neck, and in the legs.

Almost 80 percent of the blood in the body is held in the veins, and that represents the second major function of the venous system. The first, clearly, is to serve as a conduit returning the blood from the capillaries to the heart. The second involves a kind of blood bank account. When there is need for an increase in cardiac output—during exercise, for example—the veins contract and return an additional amount of blood to the heart to permit the increase in blood flow. When we stand up, the increase in pressure in the veins in the lower part of the body tends to pool blood, diminishing return to the heart.

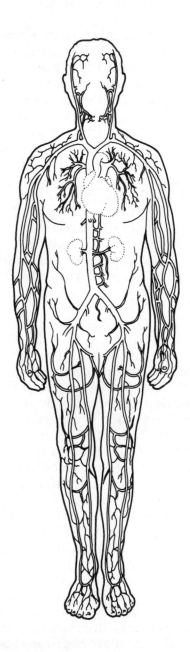

**Figure 6.   The Veins of the Body**

Every tissue that has arteries must have veins to return blood to the heart. The veins hold about 80 percent of the blood in the body.

If anything occurs to dilate the veins, the result is a fall in cardiac output, a fall in blood pressure, and a feeling of dizziness or loss of consciousness—known as fainting or syncope (see chapter 13). Everyone has experienced that feeling at times, especially after suddenly standing up. It occurs with somewhat greater frequency in older individuals because the reflex responses become more sluggish in some elderly individuals, but by no means in all. Anything that will tend to dilate the veins, such as consuming a large meal or being exposed to a hot environment, will make fainting more likely. Part of the solution, clearly, is to stand up more slowly—especially when first arising, after enjoying a nap after a large meal, or after sleeping in a hot environment.

The veins have a special feature. To prevent flow of blood backward in the veins when we stand up, or when we lift our arms or legs, the veins have valves strategically placed along their length. The valves allow forward flow, but any tendency toward backward flow closes the valves (see figure 7). If the veins become dilated, as might occur because of a prolonged increase in pressure, the dilation leads to separation of the valves so that they no longer function. As a consequence, backward flow of blood and pressure can occur, and the result is varicose veins. Because of the importance of pressure, varicose veins are much more common in women who have had multiple pregnancies—the enlarged uterus compressing the veins in the pelvis through the last six months or so of the pregnancy. In individuals who have been overweight for many years, an analogous reason probably accounts for the increased frequency of varicose veins; accumulations of fat in the pelvis may compress the veins, especially when the individual is standing.

## THE HEART'S ELECTRICAL COMMUNICATION SYSTEM

Although the function of the heart, as a pump, is very simple, important details allow this organ to perform its function normally. The heart muscle cells must all contract in an orderly sequence for the heart to act effectively as a pump. An electrical signal goes out to each cell, instructing it to contract at the appropriate moment. Within the heart are specialized fibers that represent a conducting system carrying these electrical signals. When this normal communication system is disrupted in some way, the result is a cardiac arrhythmia (see chapter 12).

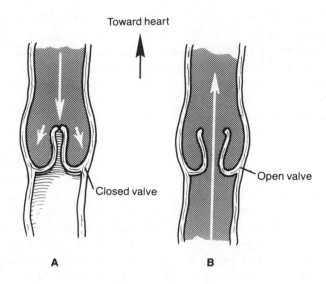

**Figure 7.   Closed and Open Valves in Veins**

Valves are located strategically throughout the venous system to prevent backward flow of blood **(A)**. When valves in the veins become incompetent, the result is varicose veins.

The resultant irregular heart contraction may be experienced in the chest as palpitations, or rapid and strong pulse. If severe, and sudden in onset, the result may be an abrupt loss of consciousness. Fortunately, benign or mild cardiac arrhythmias that require no treatment are much more common than the more severe forms; which do require treatment. Equally fortunate, where there is a need to treat cardiac arrhythmias, there are today many approaches to treatment that can alleviate the problem for most people.

## VOLUME OF BLOOD

The amount of blood in the body must be finely adjusted to fit the volume of the container, the vascular system—as, indeed, it is.

The components of normal blood also require a fine adjustment. About 45 percent of the volume of blood is made up of cells. Red blood cells carry oxygen and give blood its color.

White blood cells serve many functions but primarily are involved in protecting the body from foreign invaders. Blood platelets limit bleeding when a blood vessel is cut or injured. (See figure 8.)

The fluid part of the blood, the blood plasma, contains a large amount of protein. Also dissolved in the blood plasma are a number of minerals, called electrolytes, along with a large number of constituents—such as sugars, fats, and hormones—that are primarily there to be delivered by the blood flow to the tissues. We actually have a little more blood than we need at any given moment. That accounts for our ability to act as blood donors and represents a reserve that we can employ when we want to raise our cardiac output during exercise, with feeding, in a hot climate, during pregnancy, or with active sexual activity.

You may have read about blood doping, which represents an attempt to improve an athlete's performance by removing some of his or her blood and storing it for several weeks or months, while the athlete's body makes up the blood that has been removed. Immediately prior to the athletic performance, the original blood that was removed several weeks or months before is returned to the athlete, giving him or her a larger than

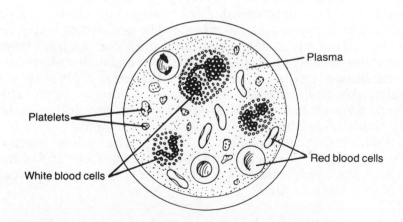

**Figure 8.    The Components of Blood**
Red blood cells carry oxygen to the tissues and carbon dioxide from the tissues. White blood cells fight infection and help make antibodies. Platelets normally plug gaps in arteries to prevent hemorrhage. Plasma is the fluid portion of the blood and contains proteins, salts, and all the nutrients supplied to the tissues.

normal blood volume and an increase in performance during strenuous physical activity. A statement made by one such athlete, that a blood-doped competitor "had a nosebleed every time he sneezed" is not physiologically accurate but is dramatic. A similar phenomenon occurs when we move to a high altitude, where oxygen is less available. Within weeks, a normal, healthy individual has increased his or her blood volume, which helps deliver more oxygen to the tissues. A similar series of events occurs in individuals who develop a disease of the heart or lungs that makes oxygen less available for delivery to the tissues. An increase in blood volume occurs that is often evident as a plum color at certain strategic sites, such as the ears, the elbows, and the knees.

Anemia is not too little blood but rather a poor supply of the oxygen-carrying hemoglobin in the red cells of the blood. There may be too few red blood cells or too little hemoglobin in the cells. That is not the same as having too low a blood volume.

## BODY FLUIDS

Blood volume is best understood as part of the body fluids. There is water inside the cells (intracellular fluid), and there is fluid around and between the cells (extracellular fluid). About one-quarter of the extracellular fluid volume is actually inside the blood vessels, as plasma volume. The volume of water inside the cells is adjusted to their content of certain important minerals, especially phosphate, potassium, and magnesium. The content of water outside the cells is adjusted to a different set of salts, especially sodium and chloride (ordinary table salt). Sodium, potassium, magnesium, and chloride in solution in the body fluids collectively are known as electrolytes.

Each of these minerals and salts works independently. Many of the consequences of cardiovascular disease, and of the treatment of cardiovascular disease, are reflected in the control of the body fluids.

### Edema

It has long been recognized that individuals with heart failure develop dropsy, or swelling. The word *edema* is now used to describe the same condition. Development of edema reflects the kidneys' retention of sodium and chloride, along with water. In some individuals, retention of salt and water might be somewhat uncomfortable, since shoes become too tight; or unsightly, since ankles swell. Anyone who has flown overnight knows the experience. With more edema than that, the result for the individual is more than uncomfortable and unsightly. Much of the shortness of breath experienced by people with heart failure and edema reflects an increase in the amount of fluid in the lungs.

Diuretics, among the most widely employed drugs today, act by causing the kidney to reject sodium and chloride and excrete them along with water. The result is a reduction in the volume of the extracellular fluid. Part of the price that is paid is that important intracellular electrolytes such as potassium and magnesium are also lost. Because restriction of sodium and chloride intake, commonly recommended as a low-salt diet by physicians, does not cause a parallel loss of potassium and magnesium, such a restriction is a sensible approach to the problem of reducing the amount of salt and water in the body. Social and cultural factors, however, made a reduction in salt intake difficult, since salt is added to many of our foods.

Of course, we can have too little salt and water as well as too much. The individual taking a diuretic for treatment of high blood pressure or edema that accompanies kidney, heart, or liver disease is prone to become dehydrated. If that person comes down with a flulike illness that includes nausea, decreased food and fluid intake, vomiting, and diarrhea—as most of us suffer once or twice a year—he or she is likely to lose too much body fluid. Under those circumstances, especially if the illness lasts more than twenty-four hours, it is wise to seek the advice of a physician. It might be necessary to discontinue the diuretics, temporarily, and even replace lost body fluids intravenously.

## BODY ELECTROLYTES

The human body contains minerals in solution in the body fluids (electrolytes), and their quantity and concentration are carefully guarded by a series of control mechanisms described later (see page 31). Cardiovascular disease, and its treatment, often expresses itself as a change in the content or concentration of these minerals in the body fluids.

When the salts dissolve in the body water, they disassociate into their separate units, each of which carries an electrical charge. The result resembles a flashlight battery. An example is ordinary table salt, sodium chloride, which is electrically neutral and forms crystals. In solution in any fluid, including body water, the sodium chloride breaks down into sodium and chloride. The sodium carries a positive charge, and the chloride carries a negative charge. In the intracellular space, the major electrolytes are potassium, magnesium, and phosphate, with a small amount of sodium and chloride. Conversely, in the extracellular fluid space, the space around and between the cells, the dominant salts are sodium and chloride, with smaller amounts of bicarbonate, potassium, magnesium, and phosphorus. An appropriate quantity and concentration of each is required for cells to function normally, and an appropriate quantity of sodium chloride (common table salt), along with the water that makes the concentration of each electrolyte appropriate, is required to maintain blood volume and a normal state of blood circulation.

Diuretic agents are among the most widely employed drugs worldwide. Thirty million prescriptions for diuretics were written in the United States last year, largely for the treatment of cardiovascular conditions. The goal of diuretic treatment is to adjust the total amount of sodium, chloride, and water in the body to an appropriate level. The price that is paid for diuretic use, unfortunately, is the frequent negative impact of these agents on other systems. Their most important effect is on other electrolytes, especially the increase in the excretion of potassium and magnesium by the kidneys. That is likely to be a problem for anyone whose diet is low in these minerals.


## THE KIDNEY AS REGULATOR

The quantity of sodium and chloride in the body is determined in part by intake and in part by the action of a number of systems on the kidney. People tend to think of the kidney as an organ of excretion, and, of course, the formation of urine is part of excretion. The kidney has a much more sophisticated job — it is actually an organ with a primary responsibility for regulation. What important components we have in the body, such as the electrolytes, depends on what we eat and what we excrete. The kidney determines what we will have in the body by determining what we eliminate. Intake of electrolytes tends to be irregular, so their excretion by the kidney becomes the important determinant of what the body is composed of.

## THE ROLE OF HORMONES

A number of forces act on the kidney to determine the excretion and retention of electrolytes and water. Among them, the action of a hormone (chemical messenger) system, the renin angiotensin-aldosterone system, is crucial. Because a number of drugs that block this system have been developed, and are showing increasing importance in treatment of hypertension and heart failure, attention has been focused on this system recently.

Renin is a hormone formed in the kidney. When released by the kidney, it causes the formation in the blood of another hormone, angiotensin II. Angiotensin II is among the most powerful blood pressure raisers in the body, acting by constricting small blood vessels. It also has a second action that is important for the cardiovascular system—it acts on the adrenal gland to cause the release of aldosterone, a hormone that acts on the kidney to cause sodium and chloride retention and potassium excretion. It is not surprising, given the importance of sodium and chloride in hypertension and heart failure, that this system is important in cardiovascular disease. For the same reason, drugs that block this system (converting enzyme inhibitors) have found increasing use in the treatment of heart failure and hypertension.

Other hormone systems probably play a role in sodium metabolism, both normal and in disease, and it is likely that we will soon have drugs that block these systems and modify sodium handling in new and important ways.

## THE SYMPATHETIC NERVOUS SYSTEM

Blood pressure and blood flow to various organs is controlled, to a major degree, by the sympathetic nervous system. Blood pressure is sensed by nerve endings in the arteries in a number of places, but especially in the neck, and that information is fed into the brain. These areas in the arteries are called baroreceptors because, like a barometer, they sense pressure. There are also baroreceptors in the large veins and atria in the heart. The information received by the central nervous system is integrated in the brain, and signals are sent out to control heart rate, contraction of the heart, and the degree of constriction of blood vessels.

The sympathetic nerves play an important different role in each organ. The sympathetic nerves to the skin, for example, are important for temperature regulation. If we are cold, those blood vessels constrict, blood flow to the skin falls, and we retain heat for reasons discussed earlier (see page 21). Conversely, if we are very warm, the blood vessels are dilated because the sympathetic nerves reduce their activity. In the case of the kidney, sympathetic nerves control blood flow and participate in the regulation of sodium metabolism by the kidney. In the case of the intestines, sympathetic nerves reduce blood flow during exercise or other activity, saving the blood flow for delivery to muscles. After a meal, on the other hand, when the intestines require an increase in blood flow, the sympathetic nerves will reduce their activity to the intestinal blood vessels, allowing blood vessels to dilate. Meanwhile, sympathetic nerves will increase activity to the skeletal muscle and other places, constricting blood vessels so the blood flow available for the intestines is increased.

### Emotion and the Sympathetic Nervous System

Many of the effects of emotions on the body are expressed through the sympathetic nerves. The pale skin and rapid heart rate associated with fear or anger are examples. If a tense emotional state can increase heart rate and raise blood pressure by constricting blood vessels through the nervous system, does it make sense that a relaxed emotional state will reverse these processes? Indeed, it does make sense. But researchers are a long way from being confident that the techniques that have been developed are adequate to induce a relaxed state routinely and reliably and sustain it long enough to make relaxation a dependable treatment for high blood pressure.

### Sluggish Reflexes

Reflexes can become sluggish for a number of reasons. Some diseases influence the sympathetic nerves and so blunt their response. A very common example is diabetes mellitus.

A number of drugs that work on the sympathetic nervous system, blocking it at one of several levels, also block reflexes. This is most commonly seen as a sudden drop in blood pressure when the individual receiving such a drug stands up too quickly. In some individuals, about one in twenty, these reflexes become sufficiently slower that a large drop in blood pressure will occur on standing, especially when standing after a large meal. The large meal requires a large supply of blood to the intestines for digestion, absorption, and metabolism of the food. If the reflexes that control digestion are sluggish, for one reason or another, a sharp drop in blood pressure, and the dizziness associated with it, will be most apparent.

## THE EFFECT OF AGING

There are no absolutes in the evolution of the cardiovascular system with increasing age.

Typically, with increasing age, the blood vessels become stiffer. They contain more connective tissue and less elastic tissue, and the result is a less compliant system. That will tend to raise the peak blood pressure achieved whenever the heart contracts. Blood flow tends to decrease in various organs as they lose tissue or atrophy. That process varies considerably. All of us know individuals in whom body muscle has been well maintained with increasing age.

When atrophy involves the kidneys, and their small blood vessels share in the process of increasing stiffness, kidney function decreases somewhat. This is not a form of kidney disease. It is for this reason that it is often necessary to adjust the dose of some drugs downward in older individuals because the drugs are excreted by the kidney and the dose that might be appropriate for a younger individual becomes too high.

In the same way, the heart muscle might show some atrophy, and the heart becomes somewhat larger, with a reduction in the peak performance it can achieve. This is an important part of the rather modest limitation of exercise that older individuals often experience. One of the secrets to maintaining a useful cardiovascular system, at least for one's age, must be sustained activity.

# 3

# The Medical Evaluation—
# A "Complete" Physical

Many people believe that tests from the laboratory, X rays, and special procedures are the most important part of a "complete" physical examination or medical evaluation. That is not correct; they are the most specific part, and the most expensive.

A medical evaluation includes your history, the findings from the physical examination performed by your doctor, information from certain routine laboratory tests—and the definition of "routine testing" is broad—and, finally, the results of special tests. Despite the many special tests now available, most experts agree that at least 70 percent of the information useful to the physician actually comes from your medical history.

## THE MEDICAL HISTORY

The medical history is information you give your physician concerning everything that could have a direct, or remote, bearing on the problem bringing you into the office. Your medical history is important for a very practical reason—it is the part of your medical evaluation that you can influence. Careful preparation of information makes it easier to establish a diagnosis—that is, identify the source of a problem—and to evaluate the results of treatment.

The medical history is obviously not the entire story of your life—if that were the criterion, we would all need to be autobiographers. What is needed is the complete *relevant* history. The excellence of a person's history depends in part on his or her physician's skill in guiding the person through the story and in part on the individual's own memory, ability to be accurate, and ability to be articulate.

Some items are routine. Examples include a record of earlier illnesses, medications being taken, family history of illness, allergies, occupation, travel, and physical activity. A general review of the various systems that make up the body is routine also. That includes the nervous system, the cardiovascular and respiratory systems, and the gastrointestinal and genitourinary systems, as well as endocrine and metabolic functions and related subjects. In short, questions will be asked concerning the function of every part of the body.

The elements in the history that are immediately relevant to the current problem vary widely. When one person has heart disease, the fact that rheumatic fever occurred during childhood might be an important clue. For someone else with heart disease, too much alcohol plays a critical role in diagnosis. For a third individual, a history of occupational exposure to some toxin might be the fact that solves the puzzle. For some people, a family history of one disease or another might be very important, whereas for another individual this element in the history is irrelevant. A recent fall or car accident might be irrelevant or the fundamental clue to the current problem.

Many physicians are now in the habit of asking questions about risk factors for atherosclerotic disease. Thus, the doctor might ask about a family history. Did anyone in the family die young because of heart attack or stroke? Is there a family history of diabetes mellitus or hypertension? Are any family members being treated for abnormalities in serum cholesterol or other blood fats? The doctor might also ask whether your blood pressure was found to be elevated on any earlier occa-

---

**RISK FACTORS YOUR DOCTOR MAY ASK ABOUT**

- Family history of heart attack, stroke, high blood pressure, diabetes mellitus, or abnormal cholesterol levels.
- Earlier incidents of elevated blood pressure.
- Smoking.
- Dietary habits.
- Lack of exercise.
- Demands and stress at the workplace.

sions along with questions about smoking, exercise, dieting (if you are overweight), and whether your work is stressful or physically demanding. A more detailed series of questions about nutrition is more common than years ago. These questions about nutrition would include whether you have made an effort to control your intake of sodium and whether you have attempted to reduce your intake of foods high in cholesterol—such as eggs, cream, marbled beef, and junk food—by replacing these fatty foods with fish, fruits, and vegetables.

A common problem brought to the physician is pain in the chest, since chest pain is obviously among the most frightening things that can happen to a person. The source of the fear is that the pain is from the heart. The pain might, in fact, arise from bone, muscle, ligament, and skin and from a variety of internal structures including the lungs and the esophagus (because of spasm, ulcer, or hiatal hernia—a protrusion of the stomach through the opening in the diaphragm, the large muscle separating the thorax and the abdomen, from the abdomen). Pain in the lower chest may be due to a peptic ulcer in the stomach or duodenum, abnormalities of the gallbladder or the pancreas, or inflammation involving the diaphragm. Questions might involve where the pain occurs and whether it moves from there to another location, the severity and character (sharp, dull ache, crampy, and so on), and events that might provoke the pain and maneuvers that might give relief. Whether the pain is continuous or intermittent is important. Intermittent pain might occur frequently or infrequently or may be changing in pattern. In each case, the medical history provides strong clues as to the source and is the most important guide, to the physician, of how to proceed.

## What You Can Do to Help

A record of any earlier illnesses suffered, the time and place of hospitalization, and the physicians that you visited can be critical. A thoughtful review of your medical history can uncover physical examinations performed for school admission or sports, as part of a preemployment evaluation, prior to obtaining life insurance, during pregnancies or evaluation for birth control, or for military service. Having each physician's name and telephone number will make it easier to obtain information. If you are on a special diet or taking medications, bringing that information to the medical interview will make your file much more useful.

A diary of events can be a very useful source of information. When did you first notice pain, shortness of breath, palpatation, or whatever your symptoms are? Conversation with others will often link it to an event: "Wasn't it right after Thanksgiving dinner last year that you first complained?" The more careful and thoughtful the preparation for the office visit, the more that can be accomplished during the visit.

Laboratory results and X rays from earlier evaluations can also be helpful. The best way to guarantee that the results of tests, X rays, and electrocardiograms performed earlier reach the physician's office at the same time as your first visit or consultation is for you to bring them in at the time of the visit. This involves doing some homework, and perhaps some running around, but it does save time and money.

The information your doctor has is critical. Far too few of us have adequate information on the medical histories of our families. How many of us know the cause of death of our parents, our grandparents, and other close family members? How many know whether relatives still alive are currently under treatment for some condition or have been treated for one? A record of this information, obtained by chatting with multiple family members and preparing a summary, can be a very useful addition to your personal file and to your doctor's office files and can reduce the time and cost required to establish a diagnosis.

## THE PHYSICAL EXAMINATION

The physical examination—inspection, palpation, percussion, and auscultation—is the next most important step in the evaluation process.

*Inspection* means "looking." The training process for the physician involves learning to look for telltale clues. Swelling in the neck or a blue tinge to the lips and the nail bed of the fingers may provide an important clue. The swelling in the neck may have occurred so gradually that no one has noticed it but can connote an enlarged thyroid gland as the cause of the problem. As Sherlock Holmes, the great "inspector," pointed out, "Anyone can look, but seeing has to be learned."

*Palpation* means "touching." The physician employs touch to detect differences in temperature; the pulses; the vibrations at the surface of the body reflecting events deeper in the body; the size of organs in the abdomen, along with their position

**BEFORE SEEING YOUR DOCTOR . . .**

1. Make notes on the medical conditions of close family members—including causes of death, where applicable.
2. Collect your own personal history—earlier illnesses, treatments, and hospitalizations. Make a record that includes physicians you have consulted in the past. Use family members and friends to help you remember events and dates.
3. If you have symptoms, keep a medical diary. What were the symptoms like, and *when* did they occur?
4. Bring results of earlier laboratory tests, X rays, and any other medical records you can collect when you visit your doctor.
5. Make a list of all prescription and over-the-counter drugs you take or have taken over the past year. Include dosages.

and mobility; and the presence of masses, as well as their consistency.

Percussion involves thumping the surface of the body with the finger to set up vibrations, and thereby obtain information about what lies below the surface. In essence, it is similar to sonar but primitive. Because structures containing air provide a different vibration than solid structures, one can discern information about the deeper parts in the body with this technique.

Auscultation involves listening and hearing. Most people associate the physician's use of a stethoscope as the pivotal element in the physical examination. In fact, it takes its place among the rest. Sound occurs because something moves in the body and thereby creates turbulence. (A river or stream moving slowly in its bed creates little sound. When the river reaches rocks or a waterfall, substantial sound is generated because the waterfall or rocks create turbulence in the flow.) What generally moves is either blood, in the heart or in blood vessels, or air in the lungs or in the bowel. These sounds can be heard without a stethoscope, as can be attested to by everyone who, when hungry, has had embarrassing bowel sounds (growling stomach or intestinal rumbling) evident to everyone in the room. (By the way, that sound has a name; it is called borborygmus—a useful piece of information for Trivial Pursuits® or a cocktail party.)

What is the doctor learning when he or she examines the heart by auscultation? A heart that sounds normal is not necessarily a normal heart. The sounds made by the heart can provide information on whether the valves in the heart are functioning normally, whether inflammation at the surface of the heart has created a surface that creates a rubbing sound, or whether the sounds are consistent with heart failure; they cannot indicate whether the heart is normal.

### Examining Your Blood Circulation

The taking of blood pressure and measurement of the pulse rate and regularity are familiar to everyone. Part of the evaluation of the circulatory system is the examination of the eye with an ophthalmoscope. The only small blood vessels in the body that can be seen directly are those at the back of the eye (see figure 9). Examination of those blood vessels is an important part of the assessment of high blood pressure. The physical exam of the head and neck includes a special evaluation of the color of the membranes in the mouth and the eye and of the lips. Is there evidence of anemia or of blue tinge due to too little oxygen in the blood (cyanosis)?

The veins in the neck are directly in line with the veins in the right portion of the heart. If pressure in those veins is in-

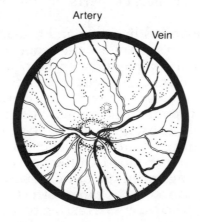

**Figure 9.   The Normal Eye**

An ophthalmoscope is used by doctors to look at the back of the eye, the fundus, which is the only part of the body in which the blood vessels can be seen directly.

creased because of heart failure or because the external lining of the heart has become very thick and rigid, it is evident as an increase in the pressure in the neck veins. They are too full. If the large valve between the right atrium and the right ventricle becomes incompetent, pressure waves from the right ventricle are transmitted back to the neck veins and are easily visible. Examination of the arteries in the neck provides information about the risk of obstruction, leading to stroke. An important structure for the cardiovascular system in the neck is the thyroid gland, since underactivity or overactivity of the thyroid can have a major impact on the circulation.

In the chest, the physician determines whether the lungs are clear. Fluid retention can result in crackling sounds in the lungs called rales. The accumulation of fluid around the lung (pleural effusion) can also be recognized on a physical examination. The size of the heart, its regularity, and sounds that indicate an abnormality of contraction or of the valves are determined by auscultation.

In the abdomen, the presence of a large liver can indicate increased blood content because of heart failure. Free fluid in the abdomen (ascites) can also be identified. Very large kidneys, due to multiple cysts, can be identified in the individual in whom high blood pressure and heart failure are due to a primary kidney disease. In the hands and feet, evidence of fluid accumulation (edema) can provide a clue to the presence of heart failure. The pulses in the arms and legs provide an indication of the blood supply to the limbs, as does the nutrition of the skin.

Taken in all, the physical examination provides considerable information—information that can be especially helpful when it has been focused by the medical history.

## ROUTINE LABORATORY TESTS

Modern technology has had an enormous impact on what might be considered routine testing. Once laboratory tests were labor-intensive, and because the persons performing them required a great deal of education and training, blood tests were very expensive. Modern technology stepped in and changed the situation. The development of instruments that make chemical measurements (the Autoanalyzer®) and automatically measure the size and number of cells of blood (counters) has reduced the unit cost enormously. For that reason, a routine battery of tests today may include measurements of blood sugar, cholesterol, and triglycerides (in search of metabolic disease); tests of kidney function (blood urea nitrogen and serum creatinine concentration); test of liver function; measurement of the electrolytes described in chapter 2 and a number of other minerals that are important to the function of various organs; and measurements of enzymes that reflect injury to organs such as the heart and the liver. One commonly employed machine performs, quickly and inexpensively, twenty-five tests on a small volume of blood. This has resulted in an extraordinary change in the pattern of medical practice, with the identification of a host of potentially important diseases possible much earlier.

Similarly, routine blood examination will also include not only the measurement of hemoglobin concentration but also hematocrit (the fraction of blood that is made up of the red blood cells) and the number of red blood cells and their average size, hemoglobin content, and hemoglobin concentration. Similarly, the white cells are routinely counted along with an index of the number of platelets, the small structures that are so important in preventing bleeding.

A urinalysis, chest X ray, and electrocardiogram are a frequent routine part of the first medical examination for most individuals—and certainly for those who are older or who have complaints relative to the cardiovascular system.

Tests need not be performed at every office visit. Tests should be ordered only when needed.

## THE SYNTHESIS

Once the information from the medical history, physical examination, and routine laboratory testing is available, the physician has to make a decision. Is all the information required to make a diagnosis and a decision about treatment available, or will some special tests be required? Clearly, the gravity of the potential problem raised by the individual's symptoms, the availability of treatment if a positive diagnosis is made, the risk of using that treatment without establishing a firm diagnosis, and availability of the special procedures will determine when they are used. In general, the increase in the number of special tests has reflected the fact that more approaches to treatment are available.

See chapter 4 for a discussion of specific procedures.

# 4

## Special Tests and Procedures on the Heart and Circulatory System

If the findings from your medical history, physical examination, and routine tests suggest that a more detailed evaluation of your heart and circulatory system is required, your physician is likely to order special tests. They will be used to establish a diagnosis, to establish the precise functional status of the heart and blood circulation, and to guide treatment. These tests have a mystique. The word *risk* may be mentioned, and thus the tests often need explanation. They are generally also much more expensive than routine tests. For these reasons, if you are anticipating these tests, you may benefit from this information: the goal of each test, the information that can be gained, how the test is performed, and what risks go along with the benefits that the test can provide.

First, perhaps it is appropriate to explain why these tests are so costly. The equipment involved is generally very expensive and has a rather short life. It is unusual for the serviceable life of major pieces of equipment to exceed five to seven years. Thus, the pieces are being depreciated, for replacement, at a very rapid rate, and substantial interest is being paid on the money borrowed to purchase the equipment. Also, these tests are very labor-intensive; their successful and safe performance involves the effects of a number of highly trained individuals whose time is expensive.

Let us take, as an example, angiographic procedures, X rays of the heart or circulation in which a dye is injected to outline or fill blood vessels or the heart so that they can be seen on an X ray. The initial capital outlay is typically over a million dollars today. If the equipment is to be replaced in five years, the yearly cost of depreciation is $200,000, or about $4,000 each week. Annual maintenance of the equipment generally comes to about 20 percent of the cost, or another $4,000 per week. With a five-day work week, about $1,600 per day is being spent before any studies have been done. If it is possible to study four patients each day with that equipment, and that is a fairly heavy schedule, the bill is up to $400 for each person before any bills for personnel or the supplies required to perform the study have been paid. Those costs are unlikely to go down. The equipment being developed reduces the risk and discomfort associated with various procedures and makes the procedures more effective, but it inevitably increases the cost.

## THE ELECTROCARDIOGRAM

The electrocardiogram (called both an ECG and an EKG) is a graphic description of electrical activity produced by the heart that is recorded from the body surfaces by electrodes that are positioned on the body so that they monitor the activity of the

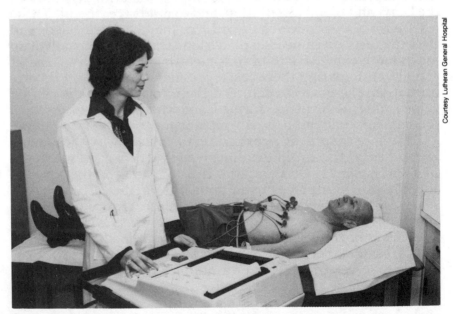

Courtesy Lutheran General Hospital

*Person having an electrocardiogram. Electrical currents produced by the heart are picked up by electrodes attached to the arms, legs, and chest. The EKG amplifies the currents, and they are transmitted on graph paper.*

heart from different directions. Information from an electrocardiogram can include evidence of earlier damage from a heart attack; the effects of abnormalities in body chemistry, especially electrolytes, on the electrical activity of the heart; and the effects of drugs on the heart. If the electrocardiogram is taken at a time that a cardiac arrhythmia is present (see chapter 2), identification of the kind of arrhythmia is extremely valuable in planning treatment. If the problem is chest pain, the electrocardiogram provides insight into whether the heart is responsible—but only if the pain is present when the electrocardiogram is being obtained.

The electrocardiogram is virtually a routine test today. The analysis is straightforward, and the cost of the equipment and analysis is relatively minor. It is mentioned here as an introduction to more elaborate tests based on the electrocardiogram.

## Stress Testing

The electrocardiogram generally gives very little information about pain in the chest precipitated by exercise if the EKG is taken while you are at rest. The electrocardiogram can be perfectly normal at rest and become very abnormal when exercise provokes pain. This is the logic behind the "stress testing," with exercise as the stress. In this use of the electrocardiogram, the electrodes are placed on the body, and the individual exercises—typically walking or jogging on a treadmill but occasionally pedaling a bicycle or using some other device—and the electrocardiogram is monitored continuously. A modern exercise test is generally designed so that the individual exercises a graded, progressively increasing amount while a responsible physician and technician keep careful track of symptoms, the work load that the individual can handle, and the impact of that work load on the electrocardiogram. Blood pressure and heart rate are also measured during exercise and provide additional information about your response to the work load. Blood pressure is important, since severe obstruction of a large coronary artery can result in a sharp fall in blood pressure, which provides a strong clue that important coronary artery disease is present. Information on heart rate is useful because individuals differ in their ability to handle exercise, and one goal of an exercise test is to achieve a certain increase in heart rate. Finally, the electrocardiogram itself provides important information concerning the coronary arteries. One important criterion for a positive test, that is, a test that indicates probability of coro-

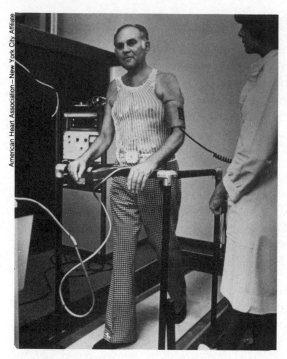

Stress testing on a treadmill.

nary artery disease, is a change in the pattern of electrical activity in the electrocardiogram.

An individual with continuing chest pain is at risk with exercise, whether or not a treadmill is involved. In such case, an exercise test would not usually be performed.

The information from exercise testing can be used in more than one way. First, when chest pain is of somewhat obscure origin, a positive test strengthens the likelihood that the chest pain reflects coronary artery disease. When there is already a strong suspicion that chest pain reflects coronary artery disease, the information from the exercise test can provide insights into prognosis (what will happen). A strongly positive stress test—that is, one that shows a very limited ability to exercise and a striking change in the electrocardiogram with very low exercise levels—strongly suggests a coronary artery obstruction that involves such a large part of the blood supply to the heart that an immediate further evaluation, a coronary arteriogram, is necessary. On the other hand, an individual who shows a somewhat positive test, but only at much higher exercise levels, often will do well with medical therapy, and no fur-

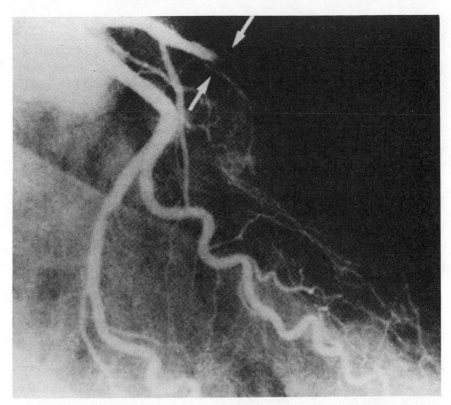

*A coronary arteriogram obtained from a man having a heart attack. The white lines represent coronary arteries that have been made visible by injecting an iodine-containing contrast agent directly into the arterial blood supply to the heart. The two arrows indicate complete obstruction by a blood clot from a major branch of the left coronary artery.*

From *Abrams Angiography: Vascular and Interventional Radiology*, Third Edition by Herbert L. Abrams, M.D., Editor. Published by Little, Brown & Company, Boston, Massachusetts, 1983.

ther evaluation may be required at that time. When individuals are not doing as well as expected on medical therapy, an exercise stress test can provide insight into just how effective, or ineffective, the therapy really is. As one example, there may be two sources of chest pain, only one of them the heart. Treatment directed at the heart, therefore, may not relieve all the pain.

Nuclear medicine tests are often performed during exercise studies to provide additional information on the blood supply to the heart during exercise (see pages 55–56).

### The Holter Monitor

A similar logic underlies the approach to intermittent, or episodic, cardiac arrhythmias. A person might have a history suggestive of such episodes, perhaps reflected in occasional fainting for no apparent cause (see chapter 13) or occasional palpitations (see chapter 12) associated with shortness of breath. The electrocardiogram taken at rest, while the patient happens to be in the doctor's office, may not reveal the source. For that reason, techniques have been developed for recording the electrocardiogram for very long intervals—twenty-four hours or more. The most commonly used device is the Holter monitor; the patient wears a recording device and carries on daily activities. Often, the physician will ask the individual to note the time an event occurs and the nature of the event—such as palpitations or pain during activity. The test does not carry a risk.

The record from a Holter monitor is typically analyzed by computer, and the entire technique reflects advances in modern technology. Solid-state physics made it possible to develop tiny, portable instruments required for continuous monitoring.

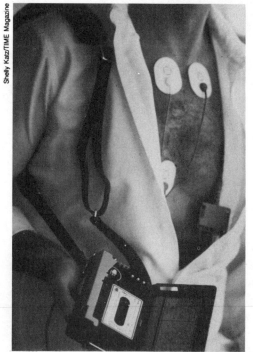

Shelly Katz/TIME Magazine

*Person wearing a Holter monitor.*

High-speed computers made it possible to reduce the work load involved in analyzing the records. If an individual has a heart rate of 80 beats per minute, on the average throughout the day, a twenty-four-hour record will provide over 115,000 beats to analyze. The computer reduces the work load by identifying the areas of the record that require closer attention. Indeed, some of the modern techniques count abnormal episodes and provide the physician with a record of their appearance.

The cost of these tests exceeds that of a routine electrocardiogram because more personnel and more equipment are involved, but the tests do not fall into the exceedingly expensive category.

## PHONOCARDIOGRAPHY

The phonocardiogram provides a picture of lines recording the sounds and murmurs that originate in the heart and circulatory system, thus adding to the information obtained from auscultation of the heart. Although phonocardiography is useful for determining the timing and characteristics of individual cardiac murmurs, it is most widely used to time precisely events during the cardiac cycle. Often it is combined with a record of the pulse over the artery of the neck to provide an even more precise measure of heart function and the status of the heart valves without the need for cardiac catheterization, that is, placing plastic tubes in the heart to help determine the way it is functioning (see pages 50–52).

There are no risks, and the test is relatively inexpensive.

## ECHOCARDIOGRAPHY

One of the most effective advances in medicine has been the development of techniques for using sound waves to provide outline pictures of the heart, blood vessels, and other parts of the body. Short pulses of ultrasound are generated by a crystal in a probe placed on the chest. The probe acts as both a transmitter of the pulses and a receiver of the ultrasound pulses as they bounce back. These sound pulses reflect off surfaces in the body and return to the crystal for detection.

Echocardiography is useful for measuring dimensions in the heart and for identifying abnormalities of the heart valves

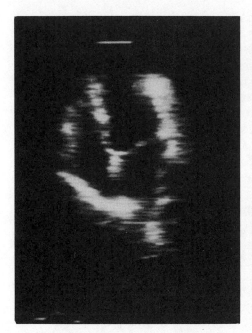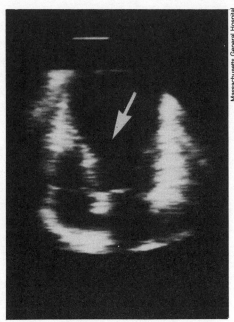

*Echocardiograms showing a normal heart* (left) *and a heart with an enlarged left ventricle* (right).

and of contraction. Again, the technique carries no risk. The cost is typically in the intermediate range. The only drawback to echocardiography is its limitation in certain areas—for example, the coronary arteries cannot be evaluated with this technique—and its dependence on the skill of the operator. Fortunately, today there are many highly skilled, well-trained operators, and this technique has moved to the forefront of modern diagnosis of the diseases of the circulatory system.

## ANGIOGRAPHY

The development of techniques that make it possible to place small plastic tubes, called catheters, in the right and left sides of the heart and in the major arteries and veins revolutionized the approach to disease of the circulatory system. These techniques provide the opportunity to make very precise measurements of blood pressure in each of these parts of the circulation and the blood flow they carry. Through the application of X rays, one can obtain pictures of the heart and blood vessels. Indeed, with high-speed cameras, motion pictures are obtained routinely (cineangiocardiography).

The term *noninvasive* has been applied to describe the electrocardiogram, echocardiogram, and phonocardiogram because such tests do not "invade" the body. They are essentially risk-free. In the case of vascular and cardiac catheterization, and angiography, the tests are invasive—placing tubes and injecting dye involve invading the body. They obviously can produce more discomfort and must carry some risk.

Discomfort can occur at several stages of the procedure. First, it is necessary to place a catheter in an artery or vein. This is done in a number of ways, but the most common is called the Seldinger technique. In this technique, a medium-sized needle is placed in an artery or vein, typically in the blood vessels at the elbow or at the groin. The needle is in place for a very short time, generally minutes, and the discomfort is reduced by injecting a local anesthetic such as novocaine into the region. When the needle is in place inside the blood vessel, a very fine plastic or metal tube, called a guide wire, is placed into the blood vessel through the needle, and the needle is removed. The guide wire is then used to guide the catheter into the artery or vein. The tube is then advanced to the appropriate location by watching it on a fluoroscope (an X-ray machine that shows the image on a television screen). The only source of discomfort is the placing of the needle and catheter into the blood vessel. Movement of the catheter inside the blood vessel or the heart does not give rise to any sensation, since the inside of the blood vessels does not have nerves.

The injection of dye through the tube to fill the cavity of the heart or blood vessel to be X-rayed may lead to some discomfort. Some will note a warm feeling or nausea. When the dye is injected into the blood vessels in the area that supplies the muscles in the back or the arms or legs, the opening up of the blood vessels can be uncomfortable. Fortunately, some of the newer dyes have reduced sharply the frequency and severity of this discomfort. For most individuals, the discomfort is described as minor.

The major risk involves having the catheter damage an already damaged area in an artery so that a blood clot forms. The complication caused by a clot depends on where the clot goes. If the X rays involve the arteries to the brain, a clot could cause a small stroke. Most clots that do form simply disappear into the bloodstream without causing any overall problem. A second problem is a bruise at the site of the inserted catheter in the groin, which can be large and rather uncomfortable. The frequency of these complications, fortunately, is very low.

Recent estimates suggest that about one person in a thousand having one of these tests is at risk of a substantial adverse reaction. With improvements in the catheter materials, the dyes, and the technique of the individuals performing the tests, the complication rate has gone down.

These are expensive tests. They use the most expensive equipment and a large number of expensive personnel. On the other hand, the development of these tests has made it possible for modern surgery to aid in attacking diseases of the heart and blood vessels. These approaches clearly qualify as a miracle of modern medicine.

The ability to place catheters and inject dye provides the surgeon with a road map so that the surgical procedures can be planned precisely. Also, catheters have been modified so that special measuring devices can be mounted on or close to the tip for the very precise measurement of pressure in localized areas or for the local measurements of sound generated in the heart. Other special catheters make it possible to record the electrocardiogram directly in points of the heart to localize sources of abnormal electrical activity and thus arrhythmias. Indeed, specialized catheters have been developed to remove the source of the abnormal electrical activity. With another modification of the catheter, biopsy (taking a small piece of tissue to examine under a microscope) of the heart can be made and thus more precise diagnosis of diseases of the heart muscle, which can lead to more specific therapy.

## ANGIOPLASTY AND VALVULOPLASTY

Finally, small balloon-tipped catheters have been developed that can be passed into blood vessels, or into calcified heart valves, and used to dilate these areas and reverse partial obstruction. This technique, percutaneous transluminal angioplasty, or valvuloplasty, is one of the more dramatic new advances in the treatment of disease of the heart vessels and heart valves. The catheter is placed in the blood vessel through a puncture of the skin that does not require surgery. The balloon-tip of the catheter is placed in the strategic location through the lumen, the central hollow bore of the blood vessel. The blood vessel is repaired by inflating the balloon to a predetermined size and pressure, again without the need for surgery (see figure 10). For valvuloplasty, of course, it is a heart valve that is repaired (see figure 11). This technique, developed by a Swiss cardiologist in the late 1970s, was considered a research procedure until recently.

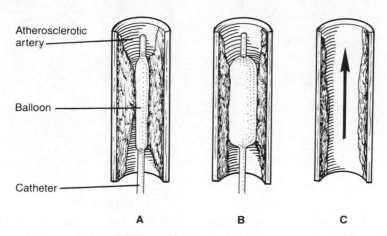

**Figure 10. Percutaneous Angioplasty**

A catheter with a balloon mounted on it has been placed in the narrowest part of the artery **(A)**. With inflation of the balloon, that narrowing has been reversed **(B)** so that free forward flow of blood is possible **(C)**.

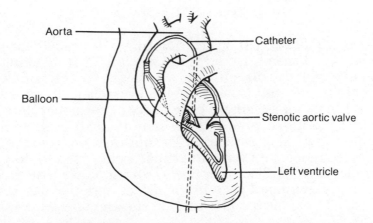

**Figure 11. Percutaneous Balloon Valvuloplasty**

A catheter has been placed in the left ventricle, and the balloon is situated in the aortic valve. Inflation of the balloon opens the stiff, stenotic, partially obstructed valve, allowing free forward flow of blood. In this way, a major operation to open or replace the aortic valve is avoided.

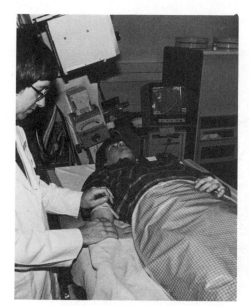 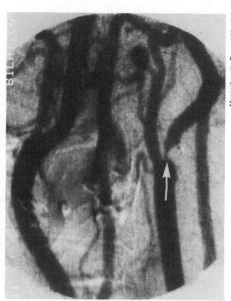

Left: *A physician preparing to insert a thin tube into an arm vein as a first step in digital subtraction angiography.*
Right: *A digital subtraction angiogram of the principal neck arteries showing a serious narrowing.*

## DIGITAL SUBTRACTION X RAY

The major drawback of arteriography, described earlier, involves the discomfort and risk associated with placing tubes and injecting dye directly into arteries. A recent, and developing, technique for visualizing blood vessels is digital subtraction. The major advantage of this technique is that the dye can be injected into a vein, rather than into an artery, so the discomfort and risk are reduced. The information from the X rays is stored in a computer, rather than being used to develop X-ray film directly. The computer is able to make a picture with much greater detail than in the direct X ray, which makes it feasible to see the blood vessels in sufficient detail that a diagnosis can be made.

This is another technique that has been evolving rapidly because of improvements in the X-ray apparatus and the computer support. It has become a rather good technique in certain bodily locations, especially for visualizing, or imaging, the arteries in the neck and to the limbs. On the other hand, the motion associated with rhythm of the heart and the complex arrangement of blood vessels in the abdomen have made it somewhat less successful for those areas. However, substantial advances have been made recently, and it is possible that this new approach will reduce the frequency with which invasive arteriography will be required.

The obvious advantages are a sharp reduction in risk and discomfort. The expense, unfortunately, is not reduced as much because the equipment required is very sophisticated and very expensive.

## TESTS BASED ON ISOTOPES (NUCLEAR MEDICINE)

There is an important alternative to the X ray for forming images of the heart and blood vessels. If one injects an appropriate radioactive material (radioisotope) into the bloodstream, the movement of that material through the circulatory system and its accumulation in various areas can be measured. Depending on what the radioactive material is attached to, various kinds of information can be gleaned through a noninvasive, and, therefore, extremely low-risk, test.

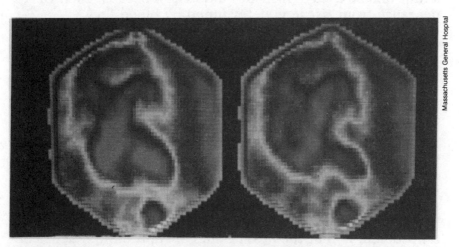

Massachusetts General Hospital

*With these nuclear medicine images that show a heart most filled with blood* (left) *and fully contracted* (right), *the physician can assess the size and the function of the ventricles and the atria.*

The radioactive material can be used to distinguish proteins or red blood cells, for example, so that they can be detected with appropriate instruments in the bloodstream. The radioisotope can be used to locate areas in which blood flow is sharply reduced and to assess the working of the heart through examining the amount of blood and its motion in the heart. This approach can be employed to detect emboli (blood clots) that go to the lung. When one injects an appropriate isotope intravenously, the area that has been blocked shows up as having a poor delivery of the isotope. If red blood cells are tagged with an isotope, they can be used to form an image of the chambers of the heart to examine the way the heart contracts and determine the fraction of blood that is pumped from the ventricle with each contraction.

Some isotopes have great attraction for portions of the heart, so their delivery to the heart can be measured as an index of blood flow to the heart in a patient who might have coronary artery disease. One isotope commonly used today is radioactive thallium. One can develop an image of the heart during exercise after injecting thallium and see which areas have a poor blood supply. Different isotopes have been used to identify damaged areas of the heart after a heart attack (myocardial infarction).

Other isotopes can be injected directly into the tissue of a limb and be used to measure blood flow because their disappearance from tissue is determined by blood flow.

These tests are not invasive and therefore carry a very low risk. They are generally not uncomfortable. Their cost is intermediate between the other noninvasive tests and angiography.

## COMPUTED AXIAL TOMOGRAPHY

The CAT scan, which is used widely for looking at structures in the head, chest, and abdomen, has revolutionized modern medicine in many areas. Indeed, it is impossible to imagine practicing medicine without the availability of a CAT scan. On the other hand, at the moment, computer tomography has not had as large an impact on disease of the heart. The fundamental problem is that the heart is in constant motion as it contracts and relaxes. Methods have been developed for using computed tomography to study the heart as it moves, but the cost of such instruments has been extraordinarily high, and they have been used in only highly specialized centers and largely

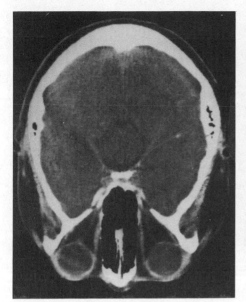 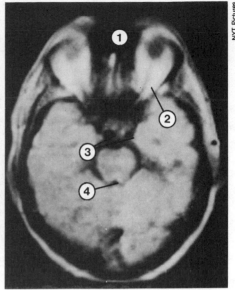

NYT Pictures

Left: *Image from a CAT scan.*
Right: *Detailed image produced by nuclear magnetic resonance, a new technique. Shown are (1) olfactory nerves, (2) an optic nerve, (3) internal carotids, and (4) a canal connecting ventricles.*

for research purposes. Another reason is the development of nuclear magnetic resonance, as described below, an approach that is likely to have a very large impact on future diagnosis of heart and blood vessel disease.

## NUCLEAR MAGNETIC RESONANCE

A very new imaging technique that was derived from a basic approach to chemical analysis is nuclear magnetic resonance. When a person is placed on a table and exposed to a strong magnetic field, some of the electrolytes that carry an electrical charge are lined up in the magnetic field, the way iron filings line up when in the field of a magnet. If a radio signal is passed through that field, the lined-up molecules send out a signal that is characteristic of the tissue that is being visualized and that can be measured. Remarkable images of parts of the body can be made. A major advantage of this approach is that no X rays

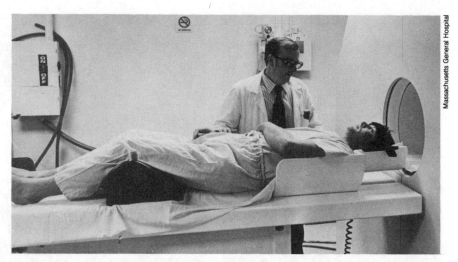

Massachusetts General Hospital

*Person being prepared for a nuclear magnetic resonance (NMR) imaging test.*

are involved, so there is no radiation hazard. The equipment is extraordinarily expensive, so the costs of doing studies are very great. The development of this technique is at its infancy, and the technique is likely to be much more important and widely available in the very near future.

# 5

## High Blood Pressure

One in every five adults in the United States has high blood pressure, or hypertension. This disorder ranks with arthritis as the most frequent chronic problem that brings people to the doctor's office. In fact, the average physician—whether a cardiologist, general internist, or family practitioner—sees every month between fifty and a hundred people with high blood pressure.

As stated earlier, the heart is a pump. Each time the heart contracts, it squeezes two to three ounces of blood into the large arteries that lead to every organ. The arteries are already full, and forcing more blood into them raises the pressure inside them. While the heart then relaxes, and refills with blood prior to the next contraction, the blood that has been squeezed into the arteries is running off into the millions of tiny, delicate capillaries that supply each organ. This blood flow, delivered to the capillaries, provides oxygen, glucose, and the various nutrients normally delivered by blood flow to each organ. As the blood runs off into the capillaries, the pressure in the arteries falls, to be raised again by the next contraction of the heart.

Because the contraction of the heart is called systole, the pressure rise that occurs when the heart contracts is known as systolic blood pressure. The interval after contraction, when the heart relaxes and refills with blood and when pressure falls in the large arteries, is called diastole. (See figure 12.) The lower pressure in the arteries at the end of diastole is known as diastolic blood pressure.

Blood pressure is reported as two numbers. If your systolic blood pressure is 125 and your diastolic blood pressure is 80, your blood pressure is 125 over 80, written 125/80. The units are in millimeters of mercury (mmHg) as a convenient device.

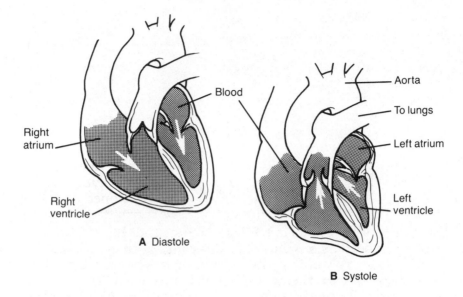

**Figure 12.   The Heart in Diastole and in Systole**

In diastole **(A)**, the atria and the ventricles relax and are filled with blood. During systole **(B)**, the atria and the ventricles contract and drive blood forward. Blood from the right ventricle is pushed through the pulmonary artery to the lung capillaries, and blood from the left ventricle is pushed into the aorta and its major branch arteries.

A systolic pressure of 125 mmHg means that, at its peak, the pressure in the arteries is just that pressure sufficient to raise a column of mercury in a glass tube against gravity by 125 millimeters.

## MEASURING BLOOD PRESSURE

A number of ways can be used to measure blood pressure. Direct measurement of pressure requires that a needle be placed in an artery. The familiar cuff placed around the arm provides a convenient and comfortable alternative way of measuring blood pressure (see figure 13). First, the cuff is inflated to a pressure well above systolic, thereby compressing the artery and preventing blood from reaching the arteries in the arm. Then, the air pressure in the cuff is allowed to fall very gradually, while the person taking the blood pressure listens to an artery below the cuff with a stethoscope. When air pressure in the cuff has fallen to the point that the blood pressure, at its peak, succeeds in forcing a small amount of blood past the cuff, the systolic blood pressure has been found. A soft "whooshing" noise can be heard through the stethoscope.

As cuff pressure continues to fall, it reaches a point where a muffled sound appears between each systolic pulse because blood also is able to pass through the artery under the cuff as the heart relaxes. At this point, the pressure in the cuff is equivalent to diastolic blood pressure. With a little practice, anyone can measure his or her own blood pressure or anyone else's. A number of inexpensive devices have been developed that simplify that measurement; some provide a printed record of the blood pressure.

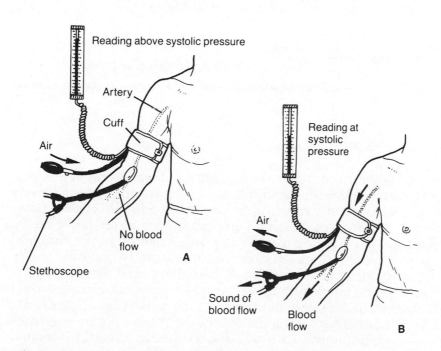

**Figure 13. Measuring Blood Pressure**

The air pressure in the cuff on the upper arm has been inflated to a pressure well above systole **(A)**. There is no flow to the artery below the cuff and no sound transmitted to the stethoscope. In **(B)**, the air pressure has been allowed to leak from the cuff until the pressure shown on the gauge exactly equals systolic blood pressure. At that point, blood spurts into the artery beyond the cuff at the peak pressure of systole and creates a sound that can be heard through the stethoscope.

$$\text{DIASTOLIC HIGH BLOOD PRESSURE} = \frac{\text{systolic blood pressure}}{\text{above 90 mmHg}}$$

Often caused by spasms of the smallest arteries, creating resistance to the flow of blood to the capillaries.

### SYSTOLIC HIGH BLOOD PRESSURE

Often caused by stiffening of the large arteries, creating the need for more pressure to pump the usual volume of blood into them.

SYSTOLE  – The heart *contracts*, squeezing blood into the arteries.

DIASTOLE – The blood in the arteries flows into the tiny capillaries.
The heart *relaxes* and refills with blood.

$$\text{Your blood pressure} = \frac{\text{systolic}}{\text{diastolic}} \quad \text{(should be 90 mmHg or under)}$$

## False High Blood Pressure

In some circumstances, the indirect measurement of blood pressure made with the cuff is not accurate and gives a falsely high reading. Only recently has the reason for this been recognized, and it is particularly important for older individuals. Some people develop a stiffening or hardening of the brachial artery (the artery in the arm that is normally compressed by the cuff) with advancing age. Such a hardened artery may require much more cuff pressure to become compressed than does a normal, elastic blood vessel. Because this occurs quite frequently in older persons, especially those in their seventies and over, attempts to lower blood pressure to the "normal range" actually produce rather low blood pressure and a number of symptoms in the person being treated. This is one of the reasons the treatment is thought to produce more side effects in older individuals.

If you are over the age of seventy and attempts at treating high blood pressure have produced symptoms suggesting too low a blood pressure, such as feeling faint or dizzy when standing up, it is worthwhile to ask your physician whether you might have false hypertension.

### Body Mechanisms for Increasing Blood Pressure

The body mechanisms responsible for increasing blood pressure are only occasionally clear. The mechanisms responsible for raising blood pressure in some of the less common forms, associated with diseases of the kidney and of the adrenal gland, are understood to a certain extent. But in 95 percent of cases of hypertension, the situation is not clearly understood.

In most people, an elevated blood pressure reflects an increase in the resistance to the flow of blood from the large arteries to the tiny capillaries, a difficulty caused by spasm of the very smallest arteries, the arterioles. One current idea as to why this resistance to blood flow is increased reflects the possibility that the cause is the use of too much sodium chloride (table salt)—especially when the body has a particular inability to handle sodium normally. Other theories place the problem in the nervous system, in the adrenal glands, or elsewhere in the kidneys. For most doctors, most of the time, the

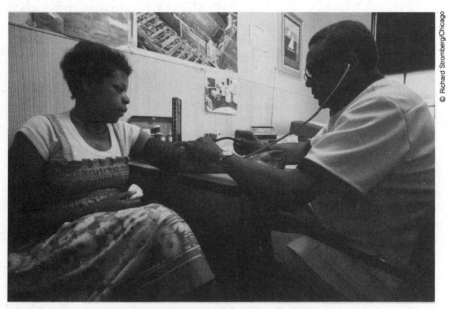

© Richard Stromberg/Chicago

*A physician obtaining a blood pressure reading.*

mechanisms responsible for high blood pressure are less important than the ability to treat it.

Physicians can treat hypertension effectively. Much treatment of high blood pressure involves a kind of "shopping around" among the available agents. The future looks bright. Physicians will do a much better job of choosing specific treatments for specific individuals when they understand the mechanisms causing the high blood pressure and can provide each person with a treatment that has been tailored to his or her individual need.

## "Normal" Blood Pressure

When physicians think about what is "normal," they are often thinking statistically—about any characteristic shared by 95 percent of the population. But, when a condition is harmful and unhealthy, causing symptoms and shortening lives, then it can be called "abnormal" in a more practical sense. High blood pressure is a case in point. Over 20 percent of the American population has high blood pressure; a statistical definition based on 5 percent does not apply. Studies on large numbers of individuals have made it clear that the higher the blood pressure, the more likely a person is to suffer damage to his or her health.

The definition of a "normal" blood pressure is somewhat arbitrary. It is apparent that a person with a diastolic blood pressure of 70 mmHg—other things being equal—is less likely to suffer an adverse event than is a person whose diastolic blood pressure is 80 mmHg. In this same way, a person whose diastolic blood pressure is 80 mmHg is statistically less likely to have health damage than a person whose diastolic blood pressure is 90 mmHg.

Most doctors agree that a diastolic blood pressure of 90 mmHg should be considered the upper acceptable limit in an adult. For similar reasons, a diastolic pressure below 90 mmHg is the typical goal of blood pressure treatment, though if it happens to come down to 80 mmHg, and is well tolerated, that is even better.

There are a number of considerations involved in deciding whether an individual, in fact, has a high blood pressure.

In our society, many more persons in their fifties have a diastolic blood pressure over 90 mmHg than those in their twenties. Perhaps as many as 40 to 50 percent of the persons who have reached their sixties and seventies will show such a blood pressure. When a large number of people who are otherwise apparently normal show an "abnormality," one has to wonder about the definition of *normal*.

There are two reasons for thinking that a diastolic blood pressure level exceeding 90 mmHg is *not* normal, or appropriate, despite the fact that it is so very common in older populations. One of the most experienced physicians in this area, Dr. Stanley Peart of London, England, has made a very persuasive argument. Individuals living in nonindustrial cultures do not show the age-related progressive increase in blood pressure that we see in ours. Moreover, as individuals move from a simple and isolated to a more industrialized setting, their blood pressure does show what physicians would call an appropriate increase with age. This observation suggests that the rise in blood pressure with increasing age in our society is not built into our biology, but rather is something acquired as a by-product of where and how we live. A compelling additional argument against considering a diastolic blood pressure exceeding 90 mmHg as normal—despite its high frequency in older populations—is the well-founded suspicion that a higher blood pressure damages health.

For these reasons, many physicians believe that it is best to think of a diastolic blood pressure over 90 mmHg as abnormal and to treat it when appropriate, ignoring the age of the patient.

## VARIABILITY OF BLOOD PRESSURE

Blood pressure changes often, sometimes with the person's mood but sometimes spontaneously. If an individual is startled or upset, the blood pressure is likely to rise. When people are asleep, their blood pressure is often normal, even if they have substantial high blood pressure.

One striking example of variability in blood pressure occurred some years ago, when a healthy individual volunteered to be a kidney donor for a sibling. The potential donor was an instructor of paratroopers in the military—an occupation demanding that he jump out of an airplane with a parachute every two or three weeks, and he had been jumping out of airplanes for sixteen years. His doctors wanted to be certain that he was healthy before removing a kidney. During one of his tests, when a needle was in an artery for purposes of a special X ray, a discussion ensued about what it was like to be a paratrooper. He obviously enjoyed his work. There was no change in his facial expression and no hint of emotional upset when he began to talk about it, but his blood pressure soared from normal to 170/110, and his heart rate increased dramatically at the same time. It appears that no matter how many times one has jumped out of an airplane, and with what success, it is an unnerving act! His blood pressure had always been normal.

Under some circumstances, with adequate provocation even people without hypertension can raise their blood pressure to moderately hypertensive levels.

This presents a problem, of course. It means that when there is blood pressure elevation, especially if it is borderline, it is not certain that, in fact, the blood pressure is always elevated and merits treatment. To make matters more complicated, it has become apparent over the past several years that having a doctor measure blood pressure—an event that is not stress-free for many individuals—can actually increase the blood pressure.

Physicians can and do deal with this problem in several ways. First, studies have shown that people, with time, get used to having their blood pressure taken. For that reason, doctors generally take blood pressure many times, and on many visits, before deciding that someone has hypertension that merits treatment, especially if it is borderline. The higher the blood pressure is, the less likely it is that the elevation is created by the stress of the measurement itself.

Sometimes even an approach to diagnosis based on multiple blood pressure measurements in the office may not be entirely satisfactory. For that reason, devices have been developed that allow one to measure blood pressure continuously, or to sample the pressure at intervals of minutes or hours, throughout the day and even the night. Much of this technology reflects a by-product of research originally performed for the National Aerospace Agency, since it was obviously important to be able to measure astronauts' blood pressure without interfering with their daily, regular activities. For this reason, many doctors interested in this problem have access to the necessary equipment and will arrange to have blood pressure measured at home, at work, and at play. At times, it may be to help the physician decide whether someone really does require treatment. At other times, the device may be used to help the doctor decide whether the medicine that is being used in treatment has been effective or to assess the duration of its effect. Most doctors would prefer to keep high blood pressure under control all of the time.

## Systolic Hypertension — What to Do About It

As individuals become older, the large arteries into which the heart pumps the blood typically become increasingly stiff, a manifestation of hardening of the arteries. As you know if you have ever attempted to blow up a balloon, the stiffer it is, the more difficult it is to expand and the higher the pressure required to expand it. Thus, as the large arteries become stiffer with increasing age, the same volume of blood pumped into them by the heart will raise blood pressure more. This is particularly a feature of systolic blood pressure.

When diastolic blood pressure is increased, the increase in blood pressure reflects increased resistance to blood flow from the large arteries into the capillaries. In the case of isolated systolic hypertension, on the other hand, the increase in pressure reflects the stiffness of the arteries.

There is every reason to believe that a blood pressure increase caused by stiffer arteries can be damaging to arteries and organs in the same way that diastolic hypertension is. What researchers do not yet have a clear answer to is the question of whether reversing systolic hypertension with medicine reduces the likelihood of injury. Because it is often not easy to reverse systolic hypertension without producing undesirable side effects, many doctors think it best not to prescribe medication.

On the other hand, if systolic hypertension is associated with another condition that requires treatment, such as heart failure (see chapter 11) or angina pectoris (see chapter 9), the treatment of systolic hypertension can be planned as part of the treatment for the other problem. This is an area in which active research is going on; that research no doubt will provide some clear answers within the next several years, along with better ways of reversing or preventing systolic hypertension.

## THE MYSTERY OF ESSENTIAL HYPERTENSION

There is substantial confusion about high blood pressure, in part because of the term *hypertension* and especially because of the term *essential hypertension*.

If physicians randomly select 100 people with high blood pressure, they will be able to find a cause for the high blood pressure of four or five of them. This group has secondary hypertension and will be described in chapter 6. In the other 95, the cause of the blood pressure elevation is mysterious. The tests that physicians can order, except for the measurement of blood pressure itself, will prove normal. These are the people who have essential hypertension.

The term *essential* is a misnomer—going back to the last century, when it was believed that the increase in blood pressure was necessary to force blood into the organs because of the abnormalities in the smaller blood vessels. On that basis, one would have thought that it would be best not to reduce blood pressure by treatment, since the increase in blood pressure was truly necessary for survival. Physicians now know (though as recently as twenty years ago, this was a matter of substantial debate) that reducing blood pressure is a very good thing to do. The term *essential hypertension* is so time-honored, and people so rarely think about what the words mean, that the name given to this mysterious process is unlikely to change.

## Tension and Hypertension

The term *hypertension* probably goes back to a French root, *tensis*, meaning "stretching or straining" and reflected the physician's mental image of the increased pressure of the blood stretching and straining the artery. Unfortunately, we often use the word *tension* to indicate mental or emotional strain. If you tie that usage to the well-known fact that being emotionally upset can raise one's blood pressure, it is clear why many individuals have come to believe that they can tell what their blood pressure is doing by how they feel. *Nothing could be farther from the truth.*

It is likely, though not at all certain, that when you are upset, your blood pressure is up. Unfortunately, the opposite is not true. Blood pressure can be elevated, and generally is, without any relation to emotional strain. Not being upset is no sure indication that your blood pressure is not up.

## Silent Injury

Hypertension is silent. An elevated blood pressure gives no clue as to its presence. It can only be found by measurement; hence, individuals generally suffer the damage brought about by high blood pressure without knowing that any damage is going on until too late. This fact accounts for the many screening programs designed to identify high blood pressure. Moreover, symptoms do not provide a daily spur or reminder to take treatment. A common problem is that patients will stop taking their medicine on their own because they "feel fine." Indeed, it is not unusual for people to feel better off their medicines than they do on them. Fortunately, a wide range of effective medications are now available, and doctors can generally construct treatment programs that are well tolerated.

## SEVERITY OF HIGH BLOOD PRESSURE

High blood pressure can vary in its severity. Most severe is a condition once called malignant hypertension, a true medical emergency requiring immediate hospitalization and immediate treatment to lower the blood pressure. Patients can be injured by the hypertension in a few weeks. Typical blood pressures in this area might be 240/150 mmHg. Such individuals often are confused or even having convulsions. They develop strokes, heart failure, or failure of their kidneys in the course of days or weeks. Treatment available since the early 1960s, however, has been remarkably effective in this area, and malignant hypertension has become both much less common and much less of a problem to treat.

At a level somewhat below a true medical emergency, the problem can be described as "urgent," requiring immediate evaluation and therapy. Admission to a hospital may or may not be required, but the evaluation is generally done in the hospital because the tests can be obtained quickly and, to insure the patient's safety, blood pressure can be monitored frequently.

Least severe is borderline high blood pressure, when the physician cannot decide at the moment whether treatment is appropriate. A decision about treatment is something that the doctor obviously wants to reach, but there is no hurry. Most doctors agree that it is better not to institute treatment until they are certain that that treatment is merited.

In borderline situations, blood pressure might be up on some occasions and not on others, and when it is elevated, diastolic pressure is, typically, below 100 mmHg. As a general rule, most doctors do not begin treatment unless they have seen blood pressure elevated at least three times in succession. The closer diastolic blood pressure is to 90 mmHg, the more difficult is the decision to treat. There is still substantial disagreement today among experts in the field as to whether borderline blood pressures should be treated, but as the available medications become safer and easier to live with, that judgment has become easier.

### Importance of High Blood Pressure

High blood pressure is important because of its long-term effects on the body. As indicated earlier, life insurance statistics and other sources of information indicate that the higher a person's diastolic blood pressure is, the shorter that person's life span is likely to be. Researchers can measure the difference in longevity between having a diastolic blood pressure of 90 mmHg and one of 95 mmHg.

Researchers can also measure a difference in longevity between having a diastolic blood pressure of 80 mmHg and one of 90 mmHg. As treatments improve, it would not be at all surprising if the goal to be achieved in treating high blood pressure moved down from the number that has been accepted hitherto, 90 mmHg.

### Danger of Untreated High Blood Pressure

What are the effects of prolonged high blood pressure? When the hypertension is an emergency, the individual can become unconscious, have convulsions, or suffer damage to the eyes. This medical emergency is known as hypertensive encephalopathy. If a blood vessel in the brain bursts, the cerebral hemorrhage produces a stroke. High blood pressure also makes the body vulnerable to atherosclerotic disease of the large arteries, and when a blood clot closes the large artery to the brain, one can have a stroke.

High blood pressure increases the work load of the heart and can lead to heart failure (see chapter 11). Indeed, until twenty years ago, high blood pressure was the most common cause of heart failure. The damage brought on by high blood pressure in the kidneys can cause kidney failure. This was much more common in the past, as a complication of the most severe hypertension in Caucasians. In some black communities in the United States, this is still a common cause of kidney damage, and it is still the most common cause of kidney failure in much of Africa.

Damage to the walls of the large arteries can lead to a bulging or ballooning of the artery wall called an aneurysm. Aneurysms can burst, leading to severe hemorrhage. A tear of the inside lining of the artery leads to a dissecting aneurysm. This is another medical emergency, in which the lining of the large artery is lifted away from the rest of the wall, creating a flap that interferes with blood flow. Fortunately, surgery now can often help an individual with this problem.

Finally, prolonged high blood pressure in the artery causes local damage, and thus atherosclerosis. In the arteries to the head, atherosclerosis leads to stroke. In the arteries to the heart, it leads to heart attack. In the arteries to the limbs, it induces peripheral arterial disease (see chapter 15), which limits one's ability to walk and can lead to loss of a limb.

Treatment, effectively employed to restore normal blood pressure, prevents many of these problems as long as it is followed faithfully. Many consider the ability to treat high blood pressure today one of the triumphs of modern medicine.

## THE MEDICAL EVALUATION

Many lay people tend to think that most useful medical information comes from the physical examination and from various laboratory measurements. As pointed out in chapter 3, most of the useful information comes from the medical history. One striking departure from this rule involves blood pressure itself. Nothing in the history or symptoms of the person with hypertension gives any clue as to the blood pressure level unless important complications have occurred—and doctors certainly want to know about high blood pressure before then. To know the blood pressure, they have to measure it.

What information is the physician in search of during the medical evaluation? One important kind of information involves the impact of the blood pressure elevation to date. Has the blood pressure elevation enlarged the heart or damaged the eyes, the nervous system, or the kidneys? What is the state of the blood vessels that can be examined?

Another broad area of medical evaluation involves additional risk factors, especially when the blood pressure is borderline and the doctor anticipates a difficult judgment as to whether to treat. Is there a history of family members having a heart attack or stroke in their forties or dying young? Does the person have a history of inactivity and of chronic overweight? Is the person a cigarette smoker? If so, how heavy a smoker, and for how long?

Is there an earlier history of some problem, such as nephritis (inflammation of the kidneys, with dark urine) that might give a clue as to why the blood pressure elevation has occurred now? Is the person pregnant or taking the birth control pill? Does the patient take medications that could raise the blood pressure (as some cough medicines or nasal sprays do) or that interact with antihypertensive medications? Does the patient eat an unusually large amount of licorice daily? Licorice can cause a problem resembling adrenal disease with persons who have hypertension. Are there associated medical conditions that can influence the decision whether to treat high blood pressure in a borderline situation?

One of the important judgments that the doctor has to make during the evaluation involves the likelihood that the problem involves essential hypertension, rather than one of the secondary forms due to an abnormality in the kidneys or adrenal glands. Because the secondary forms are so much less common, the problem is that of searching for the proverbial needle in the haystack—without any assurance that there actually is a needle in that particular haystack. One of the strong clues comes from the history of the onset of high blood pressure. Essential hypertension typically begins sometime after age thirty and before the age of fifty. An unusually early or unusually late onset of high blood pressure will point the finger of suspicion at a secondary cause, leading the physician in search of kidney or adrenal disease and a much more elaborate, time-consuming, and costly evaluation (see chapter 6).

A substantial amount of information can be found by examining the eyes of the hypertensive patient with an ophthalmoscope. The duration of the hypertension, and its severity, is often mirrored in the eyes. Changes in the back of the eye can provide a strong clue as to the stage of the hypertension and the urgency of treatment. The effectiveness of treatment often also can be assessed by looking at the back of the eye.

The physician may want to measure blood pressure in both arms, and possibly in the leg to see whether one of the large arteries between the arm and leg is blocked. He or she may choose to measure blood pressure while the patient is lying down and while standing up to see how it shifts with change in body position. In someone with borderline blood pressure levels, the physician may ask the person to lie quietly for several minutes to half an hour to see whether the blood pressure ele-

**THE MEDICAL EVALUATION**

**Clues to the Onset of High Blood Pressure**

– Do you have an earlier history of inflammation of the kidney, with dark urine?
– Are you currently taking medications that could raise blood pressure? (Some cough medicines and nasal sprays do, as does the birth control pill in some women.)
– Are you eating an unusually large amount of licorice each day?

**Routine Tests**

Urine Examination:   to identify inflammation of the kidney

Blood Count:

- serum electrolytes – to check for adrenal disease and to monitor the action of diuretics
- blood urea nitrogen – to check the functioning of the kidneys
- serum creatinine – to check the functioning of the kidneys
- serum glucose (blood sugar) – to check for diabetes
- serum cholesterol, triglycerides – to check for additional risk factors for atherosclerosis

vation settles down. Trying to find a parking place near the doctor's office in a busy area can raise blood pressure by itself!

Exactly how much laboratory testing to do generally is not a matter to be decided at the first visit. Certain tests are routine and used for everyone to provide a general baseline (see below). The more severe the hypertension, the more likely an elaborate and detailed laboratory evaluation is indicated.

## Routine Tests

Examination of urine is routine. Abnormalities of the kidneys due to inflammation will often show up as too much protein or too many red blood cells or white cells in the urine. This would provide a clue to a secondary cause of hypertension that requires additional, special investigation.

Examination of the blood generally includes a complete blood count; this is not specifically designed for high blood pressure but is part of the general medical evaluation. Certain chemicals of the blood are measured routinely. Serum electrolytes (the concentration of sodium, potassium, chloride, and bicarbonate) are measured fairly routinely for several reasons. First, they can provide a clue as to the presence of adrenal disease. Second, many of the treatments doctors use, especially diuretic agents, modify the concentrations of electrolytes in the body fluids, so it can be very useful to know what the baseline values were before treatment.

A similar situation applies to the measurement of blood urea nitrogen and serum creatinine (they provide an index of kidney function) and to serum glucose (blood sugar), especially when the person is fasting (as an index of whether diabetes is present). In both cases, treatment can modify these levels. Serum cholesterol and triglycerides might be measured as an index of an additional risk factor for atherosclerosis. If the physician finds more risk factors, he or she is more likely to treat the high blood pressure.

## More Elaborate Evaluation

A chest X ray provides a direct view of the heart, and one of the questions to be answered is whether high blood pressure has led to an increase in the size of the heart. The electrocardiogram provides similar information and is perhaps more sensitive. It also provides a reference point should chest pain occur at a later time, when the physician (and the patient) will want to know whether a heart attack is occurring. The physician is often helped in interpreting an electrocardiogram in a person who is experiencing chest pain by the availability of a prior electrocardiogram taken when there was no pain. In that way, changes in the electrocardiogram can be seen. In an equivocal or ambiguous electrocardiogram, information on a change in the electrocardiogram can be very helpful. The electrocardiogram also often provides a clue to help in the choice of therapy. For example, if the electrocardiogram reveals borderline heart block, the physician would not employ a drug for treatment that predisposes to heart block, such as a beta blocker or certain calcium antagonists (see pages 84–85).

Because enlargement of the heart can be such an important indication as to whether to treat high blood pressure, many physicians are now employing echocardiography (see chapter 4), to examine the heart. This provides a much more precise and sensitive indication as to whether the heart is enlarged than any tests previously available.

X rays of the kidney are very often employed because of the frequency with which a kidney abnormality can lead to high blood pressure. Kidney abnormalities represent the most common form of secondary hypertension. The intravenous pyelogram is a test in which a special dye is injected into an arm vein and later excreted by the kidney. The dye collects in the kidney and makes it visible. This test is not performed routinely but rather when there is some reason to suspect a kidney problem. Special studies will be reviewed in the next chapter, which deals with secondary hypertension.

## THE DECISION TO TREAT

Obviously, when the problem is a true emergency, or urgent, the decision to treat high blood pressure is straightforward. The only question is how to treat it. Fortunately there are now a number of excellent options (see pages 77–89).

When blood pressure is borderline, the decision to treat becomes more difficult. The purpose of treatment is to reduce the likelihood of any unfortunate complication of high blood pressure. But no treatment, unfortunately, is risk- or trouble-free. There is always a trade-off. The physician faces a decision as to whether the trade-off favors treatment in the individual case. The more severe the hypertension, the easier that decision is. If and when researchers find a medicine that is absolutely free of side effects, carries no risk, produces no annoying complaints, is easy to take, and is very inexpensive, the decision will become easy. At the moment, such a medicine is neither available nor in the offing.

The decision to treat borderline blood pressure elevations is made easier if associated conditions that mandate drug treatment are present. Thus, for example, if someone has many risk factors for atherosclerosis, the physician may decide that treating the high blood pressure has a higher priority than it otherwise would have. If the patient has angina pectoris (chest pain related to an insufficient blood supply to the heart), migraine headaches, glaucoma, heart failure, or some other condition that merits treatment in its own right, the treatment for that condition and for the high blood pressure can go together—this simplifies the judgment. Beta-blockers or calcium antagonists, for example, are useful both in the treatment of angina pectoris and in the treatment of hypertension.

The decision to treat high blood pressure differs fundamen-

The decision to treat borderline high blood pressure is made easier if you also have any of the following:
- angina pectoris
- migraine headaches
- glaucoma
- heart failure

tally from the decision, for example, to treat a sore throat with an antibiotic. If a physician prescribes an antibiotic to treat a sore throat, it is for seven or ten days, a limited interval. The decision to treat high blood pressure is a decision to employ medications for a lifetime. With rare exception, once treatment is started, it should be continued indefinitely. On that basis, when the blood pressure elevation is borderline and the decision is difficult, the wise doctor will often delay that decision. There really is no hurry.

## Treatment of Diastolic Hypertension

In the case of diastolic hypertension, treatment matters. To answer the question, one has to know whether people treated with a medication do better than people who are treated only with a placebo (an agent that looks and tastes like the medicine but has no drug action). A series of "placebo-controlled trials" begun in the 1960s has made it clear that the treatment of moderate and severe hypertension is well worthwhile. In a placebo-controlled trial, some of the patients receive the active treatment, and some receive a placebo, which is a pill or capsule that looks exactly like the active treatment but which contains only an inactive material. In that way, neither the patient nor the physician has any idea of who is being treated so that bias does not contribute to the result of the study.

The classic studies are those of the Veterans' Administration Cooperative Study groups in the United States, which were performed in the 1960s and whose results first appeared at the end of that decade. In the treatment of severe hypertension, an average follow-up of less than eighteen months for each patient proved that treatment was mandatory. In that short time, a substantially larger number of harmful events occurred in the placebo group. Since this powerful investigation was reported, no one has considered doing a controlled study on severe hypertension. There is simply no doubt that treatment is worthwhile.

The milder the hypertension, the more difficult it is to show a difference between a placebo group and an actively treated group. The studies take longer and must involve many more patients. In the case of mild to moderate hypertension (diastolic blood pressure generally about 100 mmHg and ranging from 90 to 104 mmHg), the next Veterans' Administration study, with a follow-up of between three and four years for each patient, showed a sufficient difference to indicate that treatment was merited. A number of placebo-controlled studies have confirmed this in the interim. Treatment for diastolic hypertension works.

## Treatment for Systolic Hypertension

As indicated earlier, the problem of isolated systolic hypertension is more complicated. It is not that physicians think that the elevated systolic blood pressure is healthy; it is simply less clear that reducing systolic blood pressure with the drugs available makes a useful difference to the affected individuals. There are a few clues from studies still in progress to indicate that such treatment will be useful, but the information has a status at the moment that leaves the medical profession in doubt. Many physicians do not believe that one should treat isolated systolic hypertension. Others believe that one should, and do so. This area remains controversial.

## HOW PHYSICIANS TREAT HIGH BLOOD PRESSURE

In the case of secondary hypertension, when often the cause is known, treatment involves either surgery or the specific medications available to block the hormone responsible. The discussion that follows really involves the treatment of essential hypertension.

There are two broad categories of approach for the treatment of essential hypertension. One involves an attempt to modify lifestyle and other factors that can influence blood pressure without resorting to the use of medications. The second involves the use of medications as the major route to controlling high blood pressure. These two approaches, of course, are not mutually exclusive, and most treatment plans include a combination.

## Lifestyle

Lifestyle changes involve, for the most part, restriction of sodium; weight loss; cutting back on coffee, cigarettes, and alcohol; and engaging in some form of meditation.

### Sodium Restriction

Occasionally one sees people consume an exceedingly high amount of salt, for cultural and social reasons. An example would be a person who often eats junk food, delicatessen items, and Chinese food. Such an individual often can achieve moderate restriction of sodium intake and can produce a gratifying reduction in blood pressure.

It is also clear, and very important, that cutting down on salt can make drug treatment easier. When restriction of sodium intake can be achieved, it certainly merits the attempt. On the other hand, most experts are currently reluctant to make a reduction of sodium intake the cornerstone of treatment for a simple, practical reason: all too often it simply doesn't work. Those relying on decreased salt consumption alone don't have their blood pressure treated adequately and have no way of knowing whether it is reduced unless they monitor their own blood pressure or are seen in the office frequently. Restriction of sodium intake, typically, is an important *part* of treatment.

It is quite clear that sharply restricting the use of salt in the diet or losing excess weight can reduce elevated blood pressure. For some people, but a limited number, that can be a very good approach to the treatment of hypertension, especially when there is only a borderline blood pressure elevation, and they are motivated to change their habits.

### Losing Weight

The individual with extreme obesity and a borderline blood pressure problem really ought to have *primary* attention paid to the obesity. As the excess weight is lost, there is no doubt that blood pressure will come down. It is an unfortunate fact, however, that modifying behavior is not as easy as we would like. (See chapter 18 for specific advice on weight loss.)

Where the overweight is modest, or the blood pressure elevation is moderate to severe, weight reduction should not be the central focus. Unless thirty pounds or more are involved, and the blood pressure elevation is mild, it is much less likely that removing excess weight will reverse the blood pressure elevation. There is also the concern that the necessary blood

The person who is extremely overweight, but whose high blood pressure is only borderline, really ought to pay *primary* attention to the obesity. As the excess weight is lost, blood pressure will come down.

pressure treatment will not be undertaken while the physician and the patient wait for the effort to lose weight to be effective. The person may disappear from treatment for the hypertension when attempts at weight loss fail; physicians know that not every attempt at weight reduction succeeds. Indeed, the frequency with which attempts to change lifestyle fail is a major problem in medicine (see chapter 18).

### Meditation
Meditation—learned from Eastern culture, society, and religion—has received considerable attention recently. It is quite clear that blood pressure may come down during meditative states. A number of studies have shown that a significant blood pressure reduction can be achieved in this way, at least for the relatively limited duration of the study. In virtually every study, the attempt to use meditation for treatment was limited to a few weeks. Most studies with drug therapy, designed to assess the influence of treatment on the natural progression of a disease, have been carried out for years. Researchers do not know whether meditation as treatment can be sustained, or if it is, whether it will change the natural course of hypertension. There is hope that meditation might be useful in the future; at the moment, though, it is still a research procedure.

Doctors do not know who can best use this approach. Indeed, in most cases, they do not know whether the blood pressure was only reduced when it was measured at the time of meditation or whether it was reduced continuously throughout the day, as is the goal in treatment of high blood pressure. Moreover, to offer someone advice to "relax," or even to teach them a little about how to relax, is not as yet a very practical approach. At the moment, it is best to consider an approach to hypertension based on meditation as an adjunct to treatment.

### Coffee, Cigarettes, and Alcohol
Coffee drinking and cigarette smoking can, at least temporarily, raise your blood pressure. No doctor would ever en-

courage cigarette smoking, and most doctors would prefer that the use of coffee be limited.

Although there is a weak correlation between alcohol intake and blood pressure when large amounts of alcohol are imbibed, the effect of alcohol is small, and a cocktail before dinner or one or two glasses of wine with dinner will not interfere with the effectiveness of antihypertensive therapy.

What all this means is that most of us would prefer not to use a medicine when a reasonable and effective alternative exists. The approach is attractive. The unfortunate truth is that at the moment there are no effective, broadly applicable, reliable treatments based on lifestyle changes. For most people, the primary treatment of high blood pressure really does mean the use of carefully selected medications. The rest is useful only as an additional measure except for the person with truly borderline hypertension, for whom nondrug measures are useful.

## Medications

As stated earlier, we live at a time when we are fortunate to have a host of effective drugs for the treatment of high blood pressure. As recently as thirty years ago, that was not true. Advances in pharmacology related to this area of medicine have been one of the triumphs of modern medicine and of the modern pharmaceutical industry.

### Diuretics

Diuretics work by reducing the reabsorption of sodium and chloride by the kidneys. When sodium and chloride are excreted in the urine, they are accompanied by water, so the body fluids are reduced in volume. Although the mechanism by which diuretic agents lower blood pressure remains somewhat controversial, this influence on the kidneys probably represents their major action to reduce blood pressure.

Diuretics were the wonder drugs of the late 1950s, when the drug chlorothiazide was discovered, followed closely by

---

Most of us would prefer not to use a medicine when a reasonable alternative exists. The unfortunate truth is that currently there are no effective, broadly applicable, reliable treatments for high blood pressure based on lifestyle.

hydrochlorothiazide and many others. Since that time, even more potent diuretics have been discovered, but none are more useful than a class of drugs called thiazides in the treatment of high blood pressure.

*Who should use diuretics?* Diuretics are effective for about 50 percent of randomly selected people with high blood pressure, resulting in a goal blood pressure of less than 90 mmHg being achieved without an additional drug. They also are employed often with other antihypertensive agents to increase their effectiveness. Although diuretics are among the earliest effective agents, their use has not yet been displaced for a number of reasons. They are effective, relatively inexpensive, and convenient to use, since they can be taken once a day. Over 700 million dollars worth (wholesale prices) were sold in the United States in 1984, to treat over 30 million people.

Doctors have a few guidelines for prescribing diuretics. Individuals in their fifties, or older, are more likely to respond than individuals in their thirties. Blacks respond more frequently than do Caucasians. Although helpful, these guidelines are not absolute.

*Side effects of diuretics.* Diuretics cause an increase in urine volume, especially when treatment is first initiated. The shorter-acting agents, such as furosemide, work very quickly. [See Appendix A for a listing of all drugs mentioned in this book — by both generic (chemical) and brand (trade) names.] (It is generally best not to take furosemide at a time when one will not have easy access to toilet facilities!) Longer-acting agents, such as chlorthalidone, will cause less trouble in this area, but because of their long action may interfere with sleep (it may be necessary to get up and empty the bladder one or more times during the night).

*The potassium/magnesium problem.* It is not only sodium and chloride whose excretion is increased when diuretics are used. There is also increased excretion of potassium and magnesium, and that may be important for the heart. For some people, a lack of potassium and magnesium because of use of diuretics can lead to irregularities of heart action, which might be dangerous (see chapter 12).

For this reason, a number of strategies have been devised to deal with the potassium problem. One strategy involves the physician and pharmacist urging an individual on a diuretic to increase his or her potassium intake by eating more potassium-rich foods, such as orange juice and bananas. However, the person who is already following a well-balanced diet is probably taking 70 to 100 units of potassium per day. (The units that are typically used are called mEq—"milliequivalents per liter of water." Potassium salts dissolve into their separate components. Milliequivalents are a measure of the concentration in solution of a simple component.) The usual supplement suggested is about 40 units per day, and a patient on a good diet doesn't need it. There is about 1 unit per inch of banana, so a typical 40-unit supplement will require eating half a dozen bananas. The same problem applies to orange juice—one needs to drink twenty-eight ounces of orange juice to get 40 units of potassium. Even the individual who loves bananas and orange juice soon tires of this regimen. Moreover those "doses" of orange juice and banana represent a substantial daily caloric burden—about an additional 500 calories. Since many are already battling a weight problem, this does not seem the best solution to dealing with the lack of sufficient potassium brought about by use of diuretics.

As an alternative, you can take potassium supplements. Potassium chloride as an elixir does not taste very good and is bulky to carry. A number of more palatable potassium supplements are available, but they still remain somewhat inconvenient in that they require multiple doses every day.

*Potassium-sparing diuretics.* As another alternative, drugs have been developed that combine a thiazide-type diuretic with a potassium-sparing diuretic in a convenient, fixed combination. The potential limitation of fixed combinations, of course, is that the physician does not have flexibility in adjusting the dose of either component. Despite that, potassium-sparing agents are widely used in this country. Indeed one of them, the brand-name drug Dyazide, was the single drug most often prescribed in the United States in 1984. A similar drug, Maxzide, has recently been approved by the Food and Drug Administration (FDA) for the treatment of high blood pressure. It has the advantage of being more reliably absorbed and thus is effective in very small doses, reducing the cost. A generic triamterene and hydrochlorothiazide is now available at 30 to 50 percent less than Dyazide. Other potassium-sparing agents available as generics are spironolactone and spironolactone and hydrochlorothiazide. Check with your pharmacist regarding availability and relative cost.

*Less common side effects of diuretics.*   Additional problems with thiazide diuretics include a rise in uric acid concentration in the blood, resulting in gout in some people. Thiazides also interfere with insulin release, so blood sugar tends to rise, and diabetes mellitus can be brought on in the occasional sensitive individual. Rash is a rare problem. A small percentage notice an intestinal upset, weakness, nausea, muscle cramps, or malaise (a general feeling of lack of well-being). In such cases, it is best that the dose be reduced sharply or that some alternative medicine be found.

Recently the very large study done on mild hypertension by the British Medical Research Council has suggested that sexual impotence can be caused by thiazide diuretics. The frequency of impotence was clearly greater in the diuretic-treated patients than in those treated with placebos. There is no clear explanation to account for why these agents may induce impotence, but it may be less common when potassium-sparing agents are employed. The onset is often very gradual, so the relation of the problem to the use of diuretics was missed for too long. Obviously if this problem should occur, alternative medicines should be employed—ideally from among those that do not have an influence on the central nervous system.

In general, the recent trend has been to reduce the dose of diuretic agents in the treatment of hypertension. Doses of hydrochlorothiazide, as a common example, often exceeded 100 mg daily; now physicians tend to prescribe 25 or 50 mg daily and add an alternative, unrelated agent if that dose does not result in the achievement of goal blood pressure. (An unrelated

---

### POSSIBLE SIDE EFFECTS OF DIURETICS

- Increased excretion of potassium and magnesium (may lead to irregularities of heart action).
- Gout.
- Diabetes mellitus.
- Sexual impotence.
- Rash (rare).
- Nausea and intestinal upsets (rare).
- Weakness, muscle cramps, or malaise (rare).

agent is a drug useful for reducing blood pressure that works through a different mechanism than that for diuretics. Virtually every one of the drugs that follow, such as beta-blockers and converting enzyme inhibitors, have an additive effect when used along with a diuretic.)

### The Beta-Blockers

If diuretics were the wonder drug for cardiovascular medicine in the late 1950s and early 1960s, the beta-adrenergic blocking agents (beta-blockers) became the wonder drug of the late 1960s and early 1970s. These agents block the action of the sympathetic nervous system on a wide variety of structures in the body, including the heart and kidneys. Precisely how they reduce blood pressure remains unclear, but as was the case for the diuretic agents, they work for about 50 percent of the people who try them.

*Who should use beta-blockers?*   The people who respond to a beta-adrenergic blocking agent tend to differ from the people who respond to a diuretic agent. Diuretics become more effective the older an individual is and are rather more likely to be effective in blacks than in Caucasians. Conversely, beta-blockers tend to be less effective for older individuals and for blacks but are often dramatically effective for younger patients. In the case of some patients in their twenties, a tiny dose may return blood pressure to normal.

In the past several years, beta-blockers have moved, in frequency of use and in importance, to a position alongside diuretics for the treatment of high blood pressure. The sales of beta-blockers in the United States in 1984 amounted to about 800 million dollars. Clearly, they are now widely prescribed.

*Side effects of beta-blockers.*   Because beta-blockers reduce the ability of the heart to increase its rate, and thereby limit total blood flow to the body during activity, many individuals taking a beta-blocker describe fatigue. For those trying to be active, and exercise regularly, exercise becomes more difficult.

Beta-blockers can be hazardous to some people. In general, it is best to avoid a beta-blocker if you have asthma or another form of chronic lung disease. Epinephrine, and agents like epinephrine, are widely used to treat asthma because they relax the bronchi. Beta-blockers act by blocking the action of epinephrine on specific receptors, preventing the relaxation of the bronchi. (Receptors are sites on a cell that a hormone or drug attach to to exert its influence on the cell.) Although attempts have been made to create beta-blockers that avoid this problem, they have been, unfortunately, only relatively effective.

For similar reasons, the person with diabetes mellitus might have a problem with a beta-blocker. When blood sugar falls, normally an increase in heart rate gives diabetics a clue that they require some sugar. In the presence of a beta-blocker, that clue can be lost. For people with peripheral arterial disease (see chapter 15), the fall in cardiac output and blood flow to the limbs can result in cold hands and feet and increased difficulties in walking. In certain cases of heart disease, a partial heart blockage can be made worse by a beta-blocker. None of these reactions reflect a mystery but rather are clearly understood in terms of chemical interaction.

Some patients describe disturbing central nervous system problems associated with beta-blockers, including changes in sleep patterns, nightmares, and depression. The more soluble in fat (lipid soluble) a beta-blocker is, the more likely it is to accumulate in the brain and produce these disturbing effects. Beta-blockers differ widely in their lipid solubility and thus in their access to the brain and their tendency to produce this type of side effect. Propranolol hydrochloride is the most lipid-soluble beta-blocker, and nadolol is the least. Switching from one medication to another might be helpful when central nervous system side effects occur.

---

**POSSIBLE SIDE EFFECTS OF BETA-BLOCKERS**

- Fatigue during exercise.
- Bronchial constriction (hazardous to those with asthma or chronic lung disease).
- Loss of cue that blood sugar is low (increased heart rate) for diabetics.
- Increased difficulty walking (for those with peripheral arterial disease).
- Potential aggravation of heart block.
- Possibility of changed sleep patterns, nightmares, and depression (more fat-soluble beta-blockers particularly).

### Diuretics Combined with Beta-Blockers
When a diuretic and a beta-blocker are used together—as they often are—their effect on blood pressure tends to be additive; that is, together they result in a larger fall in blood pressure than when either drug was employed alone. Once the appropriate dose of each is found, there are convenient combinations that simplify treatment by reducing the number of pills to be taken. Drug combinations can thus make treatment more convenient.

### Agents That Act Through the Central Nervous System
A number of drugs act to lower blood pressure primarily through an influence on critical centers in the brain. The result is a reduction in blood pressure through a decrease in sympathetic nervous system activity. Conceptually, this is a very attractive approach, but agents in this class (methyldopa, clonidine hydrochloride, and guanabenz acetate) have been less widely used because of their side effects.

A substantial percentage of people treated with this kind of agent suffer from tiredness, drowsiness, and depression—often more evident to family members than to themselves. Many people who have used this class of agent for years, however, notice a real improvement in their mood, temperament, and ability to function when the agent is stopped.

Methyldopa was once among the most widely employed agents in the treatment of high blood pressure in this country. In the early 1970s, it was recommended as the second preferred agent, after a diuretic. There are still substantial numbers of people being treated with methyldopa, many of whom have been for a number of years. Physicians rarely recommend a change of treatment for a patient who is doing well, and generally patients remain on a regimen that works and is reasonably well tolerated. On the other hand, if central nervous system side effects are a problem, it is reasonable to think about alternatives. A generic formulation is available.

### Agents That Block the Sympathetic Nerves Peripherally
Agents of this type were once substantially more important in the treatment of high blood pressure than they are now. Reserpine, originally identified in an Indian herb remedy, was frequently prescribed in the 1950s. It has a central nervous system action rather like the agents discussed above, but the depression it induces is rather severe, and now it is used only occasionally.

Guanethidine works like reserpine by depleting epinephrine and norepinephrine from body stores and by preventing norepinephrine release from nerves. Unfortunately, it tends to produce a striking fall in blood pressure when the individual stands up, diarrhea, and failure of ejaculation in men. For these reasons, it has only occasional use, generally for those with very severe hypertension for whom other approaches to treatment have been unsuccessful.

Prazosin, terazosin, and trimazosin act by preventing the action of norepinephrine on a class of receptors on blood vessels called alpha receptors. Alpha receptor activation normally causes blood vessels to constrict, hence raising blood pressure. Blocking these receptors, therefore, will tend to reduce blood pressure. In some people, there appears to be an increase in sympathetic nervous system drive—which may be responsible for their hypertension—and prazosin can be a very good choice. In most cases, prazosin seems to be somewhat less effective,

---

**SIDE EFFECTS OF DRUGS THAT BLOCK
THE SYMPATHETIC NERVES PERIPHERALLY**

reserpine: severe depression

guanethidine: dizziness upon standing up, diarrhea, failure to ejaculate

prazosin: dizziness upon standing up

**SIDE EFFECTS OF
CONVERTING ENZYME INHIBITORS**

- rash

- interference with sensation of taste

- low white blood count (rare)

- protein in the urine (rare)

**AVAILABLE AS GENERICS**

- thiazide diuretics

- methyldopa

- propranolol

and it loses its effectiveness very rapidly. Since physicians have difficulty in identifying who is likely to do well on prazosin, it has not achieved as wide use as the agents described earlier. It, too, tends to produce a substantially larger fall in blood pressure when the patient is standing than when lying down. This can produce symptoms, especially dizziness upon suddenly standing up.

### Agents That Act Through Converting Enzyme Inhibition

As beta-blockers were the wonder drug of the early 1970s for the treatment of high blood pressure, the converting enzyme inhibitor captopril was the wonder drug of the late 1970s and early 1980s. This agent and newer forms, enalapril maleate and lisinopril, act by preventing the formation of angiotensin II, which is a hormone that raises blood pressure and causes sodium retention.

When captopril was first used, it simplified enormously the treatment of severe hypertension. Patients who had required three drugs to control their blood pressure now often needed only captopril or captopril combined with a low dose of a diuretic. Doctors have found increasing use for converting enzyme inhibitors for the treatment of high blood pressure because they do not produce the annoying central nervous system side effects that plague treatment with so many of the other agents. Many experts feel that converting enzyme inhibitors will join diuretics and beta-blockers as first-line treatment.

Captopril and enalapril cause rash and a loss of the sensation of taste in a small percentage of cases, even when low doses are used. In most patients, the rash is mild and transient, but in some the rash or loss of taste is sufficiently severe that it is necessary to discontinue the use of a converting enzyme inhibitor. Whether the newer converting enzyme inhibitors will be better tolerated is not yet clear.

### Vasodilators

Because increased resistance to blood flow in the arterioles is responsible for the high blood pressure of most people with essential hypertension, the use of an agent that dilates the arterioles seems a good approach to treating the condition. Unfortunately, none of the nonspecific vasodilators currently available (hydralazine, minoxidil, diazoxide) can be used alone in hypertension. They tend to cause severe sodium retention; a diuretic, sometimes in very large doses, is always required when they are used. They also tend to raise heart rate, which can be annoying, so a beta-blocker is also often required. For that reason, their use is generally reserved for the treatment of severe high blood pressure—and with the availability of captopril, their use has decreased sharply.

### Calcium Channel Blocking Agents

This group of agents (nifedipine, verapamil, diltiazem) also act as vasodilators, but for reasons that are not yet clear, they tend to produce fewer vasodilator-related side effects than do the other vasodilators. Only one of these agents, verapamil, is currently approved by the FDA for the treatment of high blood pressure in the United States. They are generally used for the treatment of angina pectoris, but when someone with angina pectoris also has high blood pressure—the diseases occur simultaneously in about 15 percent of patients treated for high blood pressure—it is generally necessary to reduce the dose of other antihypertensive drugs or discontinue them if a calcium channel blocking agent is employed.

All the available agents are likely to receive approval in the near future and play an important role in the treatment of high blood pressure. They will probably be especially useful to older people, individuals with angina pectoris, or those in whom there is some reason to avoid the use of a beta-blocker or other antihypertensive drug.

### Generics

When a drug has been protected by a patent for seventeen years, the patent right ends and generic drugs become available. That is, other companies can then manufacture the drug. The generic drug and its brand-name counterpart contain the same active ingredients, are identical in strength and dosage forms, are taken the same way, and are just as safe. The generic, of course, has the advantage of being substantially less expensive—often by as much as 50 percent. In the United States, generics do require FDA approval, and their quality is generally good. Specific examples of a generic product not matching the original in quality do exist, however.

Because the thiazide diuretics have been around for a long time, it is not surprising that generic agents have been available for some time too. Potassium-sparing combinations are also now available as generics.

Methyldopa is also an agent that has a long history, and generics are available. For reasons reviewed above, methyldopa is not as widely employed as it once was, but a patient doing

---

**KEEPING TRACK OF MEDICATION YOU'VE TAKEN**

A useful device for keeping track of whether one has taken the day's medication or not (and which enables members of the family to provide a helpful hand, if necessary) is a weekly drug dispenser. This is especially useful when an individual has to take multiple medicines each day. At the beginning of the week, a full week's supply can be placed in individual tubes labeled *Monday*, *Tuesday*, etc. A glance then tells whether that day's medication has been taken. In that way, family members can help out, by being able to see when a reminder is actually needed.

---

well on methyldopa could consider the use of a generic. Among the beta-blockers, only propranolol, the most widely employed beta-blocker, is sufficiently mature for a generic to have been developed. When propranolol has been well tolerated, the patient can switch to a generic. Unfortunately, the beta-blockers with especially favorable features, such as a long duration of action and a reduced tendency to produce central nervous system side effects, are many years away from equivalent products.

It will be some time before generics are available for the newer wonder drugs, the converting enzyme inhibitors.

Several books are now available that describe special

---

**CHOOSING A BLOOD PRESSURE MONITOR**

A blood pressure reading taken at home can be a way of participating in your treatment. Of course, a series of normal readings at home is no reason to stop taking medication for high blood pressure! If you buy a home blood pressure monitor, make sure to bring it with you to your next appointment with your doctor so that he or she can check to be sure you are reading it correctly.

The simplest kind of monitor to use is the electronic variety, which inflates automatically. You position it correctly, press a button, and read a display. This is also the most expensive, ranging from $70 to $150 in price. If you are willing to inflate the cuff yourself, the price range goes down to $45 to $89. One problem with electronic machines is their accuracy. Sometimes they can be in error by 5 mmHg or more.

Mechanical blood pressure gauges are often more accurate. They cost less, ranging from $18 to $30. However, they also require some practice to use, as well as good hearing (to use the stethoscope).

precautions regarding drugs, information about drug reactions, and a description of how to use the medications properly. These include the following: *AARP Pharmacy Service Prescription Drug Handbook*, published by the American Association of Retired Persons and Scott, Foresman and Company, 1988 (write to AARP Books, Scott, Foresman and Co., 1865 Miner Street, Des Plaines, IL 60016); and *Advice for the Patient: Drug Information in Lay Language*, Sixth Edition, 1986, published by the United States Pharmacopeial Convention, Inc. (Order Processing Department, P.O. Box 2248, Rockville, Maryland).

### Cost of Treating High Blood Pressure

The current cost of treating hypertension can range from as little as $3.75 for a three-month prescription of a generic thiazide, to $100.00 a month for combination therapy of high doses of the more expensive brand-name products. It is generally possible to adjust treatment around side effects, effectiveness, and cost. Certainly, people should feel free to discuss cost with their physician or their pharmacist; a prudent consumer ought to "shop around" for the best price on a given prescription. Some of the newer drugs tend to be more expensive, but if they are better tolerated, they are certainly a very good investment. Depression, dizziness, distorted sleep patterns, and disturbed sexual function can be reversed with judicious selection of medications, and the investment of time and money is often worthwhile.

# 6

# Secondary Hypertension

Entire textbooks are written on the individual diseases that lead to secondary hypertension.

## KIDNEY-RELATED HYPERTENSION

Involvement is usually with the kidneys, the arteries leading to the kidneys, or the adrenal glands. Kidney involvement can be due to inflammation of the kidney itself (one of many forms of nephritis), inflammation of the small arteries leading to the kidney (arteritis), inherited abnormalities that lead to cyst formation in the kidney (polycystic kidney disease), or damage due to various drugs or poisons. (In youngsters, the latter is most common.) In older individuals, obstruction of one or more arteries to the kidney due to arterial disease is a much more common cause, leading to what is known as renal vascular, or renovascular, hypertension. Although renal vascular hypertension is uncommon—responsible for high blood pressure in no more than 3 percent of individuals with hypertension—it is the most common curable cause and so has received substantial attention. The more severe the elevation of blood pressure, the more urgent it is to identify a specific, reversible cause.

When a doctor suspects that your hypertension is secondary to some definable cause, the result is likely to be a substantial investigation in search of the cause.

### Identifying Renal Vascular Hypertension

Other than age at onset and severity of hypertension, the physician occasionally will get a clue as to the presence of renal vascular hypertension from hearing an unusual sound (bruit) when he or she listens to the upper abdomen of the patient. When the obstruction in the artery is critical, turbulence in the artery created by the blood flowing through the narrow area becomes audible.

Among the special studies for renal vascular hypertension is the intravenous pyelogram, mentioned earlier (see page 75). If there is a strong reason for suspicion, the doctor may request an arteriogram, which is an X ray of the arteries leading to the kidneys (see chapter 4). To perform that test, a radiologist places a plastic tube, a catheter, into the aorta, the large artery that leads to the renal arteries. A dye is then injected, which makes the arteries visible. This test is uncomfortable and expensive and carries a small but measurable risk (perhaps 1 in 1,000 individuals will have some damage to an artery caused by the test), so it is used very selectively.

### Treatment of Renal Vascular Hypertension

If a person has renal vascular hypertension, typically the doctor will think it best that the artery be opened or the kidney removed if it has been irreversibly damaged because of low blood flow. The artery can be reopened or bypassed by a surgeon. Surgery as an approach to the problem of renal vascular hypertension has been available for many years and is successful. But surgery carries a measurable risk and demands a fair amount of time in the hospital.

More recently, a new approach, percutaneous transluminal angioplasty, has been developed as an alternative to surgery (see pages 52–53). The procedure can be done by way of needles and catheters placed through the skin and does not require surgical exposure of the kidney and arteries to the kidney, as traditional surgical approaches do. The procedure is performed with special catheters designed with a balloon at the end that are placed directly through the narrow space within the artery leading to the kidney.

When the balloon is inflated, it opens the narrowed area, improving blood flow to the tissue at risk. This technique has been employed to reverse renal vascular hypertension with great success in many centers. Its disadvantage lies in the fact that physicians know much less about the long-term effects, since it is still a relatively new technique, and that experience and special skills are required.

For identifying inflammation within the kidneys, the physician depends initially upon tests of kidney function and characteristics of the urine analysis. When there appears to be inflammatory disease of the kidney, a renal biopsy might be used. In this test, a needle is placed into the kidney from the back, and a small piece of kidney is removed for examination under the microscope. A renal biopsy is performed if there is strong reason to believe that inflammation in the kidney is present; it is performed primarily because there now are specific treatments for some of the inflammatory renal diseases.

## ADRENAL DISEASE

A number of different abnormalities involving the adrenal glands can lead to high blood pressure. The adrenal glands lie just above the kidneys on each side. Abnormalities that can lead to high blood pressure include tumors of the adrenal and adrenal overactivity that reflect an increase in the number of cells (hyperplasia).

If the tumor is in the inner portion of the adrenal, the adrenal medulla, it tends to produce high blood pressure through the release of the hormones adrenaline and noradrenaline (epinephrine and norepinephrine). These tumors are called pheochromocytomas and fortunately are distinctly uncommon; the hormones they release can cause substantial trouble. Most are benign, but occasionally a malignant tumor does occur.

Tumors involving the outer layer of the adrenal gland can lead either to primary aldosteronism (too much aldosterone, a sodium-retaining hormone made by the adrenal) or Cushing's syndrome (too much cortisone). Primary aldosteronism is generally recognized because of a very low serum potassium associated with the high blood pressure, though that may not become apparent until the patient takes a diuretic. Cushing's syndrome is generally suspected from the patient's characteristic appearance—obesity of the face and trunk, with rather slim arms and legs; "buffalo hump" pad of fat at the top of the back just below the neck; thin skin that bruises easily; and, commonly, acne and hair growth in inappropriate places. Treatment with cortisone produces a similar appearance, which is familiar to many.

These problems are diagnosed by specialized tests involving measurements of plasma and urine concentrations of hormones. The treatment is generally surgical removal of the involved gland, though there now are medicines that will block the actions of the various hormones. These are especially helpful when the tumor cannot be removed.

All these conditions are rare, and identifying them is expensive. For these reasons, most doctors will order specialized tests only when there is a strong suspicion of a condition based on the medical history, the physical examination, or the first battery of routine tests. Since hypertension itself is so very common, the search for these relatively rare problems that produce hypertension is also common.

# 7

# Arteriosclerosis — Atherosclerosis and "Hardening of the Arteries"

Arteriosclerosis, including all the abnormalities of arteries that result in thickening and hardening, is the most common source of illness in Western society.

Atherosclerosis is one among several specific forms of arteriosclerosis and the most frequent and serious problem. The microscope has made the hallmark of atherosclerosis visible — its content of fatty (lipid) material, especially cholesterol. Cholesterol is one form of body fat. There are many different fats that have different chemical structures.

Over seventy years ago, Russian investigators interested in the influence of diet on cardiovascular disease modified the diet of rabbits, who normally eat a vegetarian diet and who normally have a very low level of blood lipids and cholesterol. When fed animal fats, the rabbits quickly developed atherosclerosis. It was soon discovered that feeding them pure cholesterol was sufficient to bring on the disease. Since that time, atherosclerosis has been successfully induced in virtually all species by manipulation of the diet.

This approach not only reinforced the importance of diet in the development of atherosclerosis — a concept still alive and vigorous today — but also made it possible to dissect the complex factors that interplay in the development of atherosclerosis. The problem is not simply the presence of too much fat, and too much cholesterol, in the diet. For example, it was shown that combining a much lower amount of cholesterol with an increased amount of triglycerides (another form of fat) would also result in atherosclerosis.

Administration of estrogen reversed the disease in birds,

even when the birds remained on a high-fat, high-cholesterol diet. This was the first observation to provide hope that treatment might be helpful and insight as to why atherosclerosis occurs earlier and with greater severity in men.

## THREE CONCLUSIONS ABOUT ATHEROSCLEROSIS

By the early 1950s, the vast experimental evidence that had accumulated led to three fundamental conclusions. First, atherosclerosis is both a nutritional and a metabolic disease. Long-term intake of diets high in fat and cholesterol, leading to an increase in their blood levels, is a key factor in its cause. Second, the disease has other causes in addition to diet. Investigation into these factors continues today. Third, and perhaps most important, atherosclerosis is not only preventable but also potentially reversible, depending on its severity and its extent.

## THE ONSET OF VASCULAR DAMAGE

Although the impact of atherosclerosis in terms of heart attack, stroke, peripheral arterial disease, and obstruction of the arteries to the kidneys and elsewhere typically begins to show up when individuals reach their forties, it has long been recognized that evidence of vascular injury (see figures 14 and 15) is present much earlier in life. During the Korean War, for example, a disturbing percentage of young men killed in action showed evidence of coronary artery disease. More recently, and even more disturbing, a very important observation was made. In the Bogalusa area of Louisiana, a large number of youngsters were examined for risk factors for high blood pressure and for hardening of the arteries while they were still in their early school years. They were then followed for a number of years. Tragically, a number came to early postmortem examination because of accidents or suicide. What became clear from that study was that risk factors—discussed in greater detail below—including elevated blood pressure, abnormal blood lipids, and heredity were inducing more advanced arterial disease despite the fact that these persons were still in their teens or early twenties. These risk factors produce their damage very gradually, over many years. The ability to reverse this vascular damage, then, becomes very important.

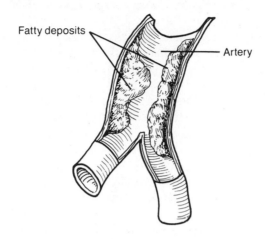

## Figure 14.   Fatty Deposits That Clog Arteries

The deposits are sufficient to almost block the artery on their own.

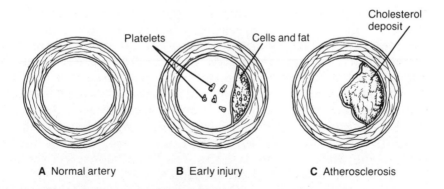

## Figure 15.   Progression of Atherosclerosis

With early injury **(B)**, there is an increase in the number of cells in the inner portion of the artery, and platelets tend to adhere to that area. With progression of atherosclerosis **(C)**, there is a deposit of cholesterol and formation of a progressively larger plaque. It is not unusual for a blood clot to deposit on the plaque.

## INVESTIGATING THE RISK FACTORS

In animal studies, it was quite clear that removing the offending element in the diet or adding appropriate hormones such as estrogen would reverse the damage of arteriosclerosis. Indeed, the estrogen given to birds would reverse the disease even when the offending diet was continued. More recently, it was shown that for animals with coronary artery disease caused by diet, a systematic exercise program would arrest the disease, and perhaps reverse it. Exercise had this effect despite continued dietary aggravation of the disease.

Perhaps the most dramatic early evidence in humans came from examination of the significant effect of altered diet learned from the mortality experience during World War II. Despite the horror of war, there was a sharp decline in death rates from atherosclerosis that occurred in Holland, Leningrad, and the Scandinavian countries. In each case, the deprivation associated with war prevented heart attacks. To the extent that the horrors of siege, occupation, and war must have increased psychic and emotional tension, the effects were more than reversed, it appears, by the reduction in intake of calories and fats. More rigorous evidence follows.

The intriguing findings from these early studies were confirmed and extended by long-term epidemiological studies in representative samples of the United States population. Factors associated with an increased risk of atherosclerotic heart disease in middle-aged men included an increase in serum cholesterol, high blood pressure, obesity, diabetes mellitus, hypothyroidism, heavy smoking, and a strong family history of premature vascular disease. All these factors were recognized and, indeed, measured by the early 1960s. At that time, it was suspected that sedentary living and psychological stress might be implicated, but clear-cut evidence was not available.

Since that time, continued investigation has led to clearer insights into the risk factors in people's lives. These insights include details of metabolism that lead to atherosclerosis and will soon have an impact on treatment.

A major long-term study was instituted in the 1950s in Framingham, Massachusetts. By thirty years ago, it was possible to measure the role of risk factors. For example, it was found that hypercholesterolemia was associated with a three- to six-fold increase in the risk of coronary artery disease. It was also found that the higher the serum cholesterol (that is, the concentration of cholesterol in the blood serum), the greater the risk. There was some difficulty in deciding what a normal serum cholesterol concentration really is. For example, in 1960, Dr. Jeremiah Stamler, a leading figure in the field, said, "These data have additional significance because they illuminate a long-standing problem, that of proper standards for normal serum cholesterol. It is certainly sound to regard 225 milligrams of cholesterol in each 100 milliliters of plasma as the upper limit of normal; further work might indicate the validity of accept-

---

### THE FRAMINGHAM HEART STUDY

The height of each bar represents the number of men forty years of age who will develop cardiovascular disease in an eight-year period among 1,000 men studied. Thus, for example, the 100 level represents a 10 percent likelihood. You will note that at the far right there was a likelihood of over 70 percent that a man would develop cardiovascular disease in eight years if he had a high systolic blood pressure, had a high blood cholesterol level, had high blood sugar, was a cigarette smoker, and had a large left ventricle.

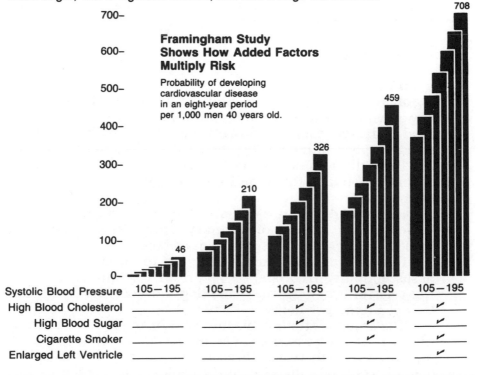

**Framingham Study Shows How Added Factors Multiply Risk**

Probability of developing cardiovascular disease in an eight-year period per 1,000 men 40 years old.

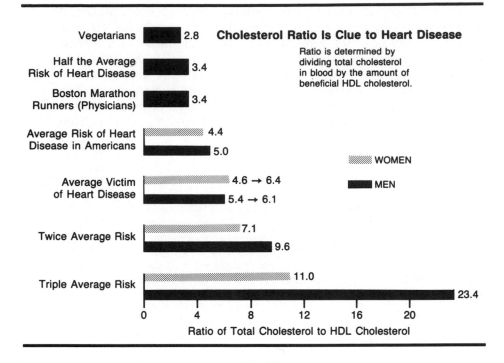

Vegetarians — 2.8

**Cholesterol Ratio Is Clue to Heart Disease**

Ratio is determined by dividing total cholesterol in blood by the amount of beneficial HDL cholesterol.

Half the Average Risk of Heart Disease — 3.4

Boston Marathon Runners (Physicians) — 3.4

Average Risk of Heart Disease in Americans — 4.4 / 5.0

▨ WOMEN
■ MEN

Average Victim of Heart Disease — 4.6 → 6.4 / 5.4 → 6.1

Twice Average Risk — 7.1 / 9.6

Triple Average Risk — 11.0 / 23.4

Ratio of Total Cholesterol to HDL Cholesterol

0  4  8  12  16  20

ing an even lower level." Dr. Stamler would surely agree that few of us would accept that serum concentration in a middle-aged individual today, and many experts would prefer to assign the upper limit of normal to a value below 200 milligrams per 100 milliliters of plasma. The fact is that physicians can do more about it today and will be able to do even more tomorrow.

High blood pressure was also found to induce a three- to six-fold increase in risk of coronary artery disease. Again, the higher the pressure, the greater its effect.

Obesity was associated with a two- to three-fold increase in susceptibility to coronary artery disease. A similar influence was seen for heavy cigarette smoking and a positive family history of premature coronary artery disease.

The accumulation of this information made it possible, by the early 1960s, to examine the influence of combinations of factors. Thus, only two or three among a hundred middle-aged men with normal values for serum cholesterol, blood pressure, and weight would have an event related to coronary artery disease in the next ten years in the Framingham study. In contrast, among a hundred men in whom any three of these factors were abnormal, thirty to forty would have such an event in the next ten years.

These data mean that a forty-five-year-old American male who is free of clinical evidence of coronary artery disease and of all risk factors has only about one chance in twenty or thirty of having a heart attack or of developing angina pectoris before the age of sixty-five. His counterpart with two risk-increasing factors has one chance in two, and if three risk factors are present, the odds increase to two chances in three between the ages of forty-five and sixty-five. The greater the number in terms of precisely how high the serum cholesterol or blood pressure is, or how many cigarettes smoked, or how overweight the individual is, the greater the risk. Fortunately, examination of the list shows that individuals can do something about every aspect, except the strong family history. Equally fortunately, we are coming to recognize how a strong family history can have its impact and thus influence the course through interrupting the responsible mechanisms. Although we

**INTERRELATIONSHIP BETWEEN RISK FACTORS AND CARDIOVASCULAR DISEASE**

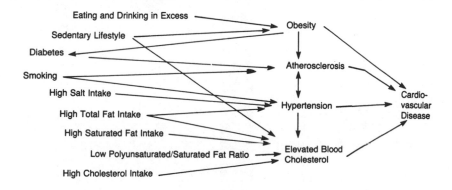

Other Risk Factors: Stress, Age, Genetics, Poor Nutrition

cannot choose our grandparents, we can choose to reduce the impact of inheritance on our bodies.

In his review article in 1960, Dr. Stamler pointed out that atherosclerotic disease, particularly coronary heart disease, is the major public health problem in the United States and in other economically developed countries. Clearly, this was a problem for the middle-aged by the early 1960s. Among 1,000 men at age forty-five, about 100 would be expected to die by the age of fifty-four. Of those 100 deaths, over one-third would come from heart disease that could be prevented or reversed. To quote Dr. Stamler, "This is our number one epidemic disease at mid century. There is no reason to believe that a policy of watchful waiting, judicious neglect, therapeutic nihilism

**COMBINATION OF RISK FACTORS THAT INCREASES DANGER OF HEART DISEASE**

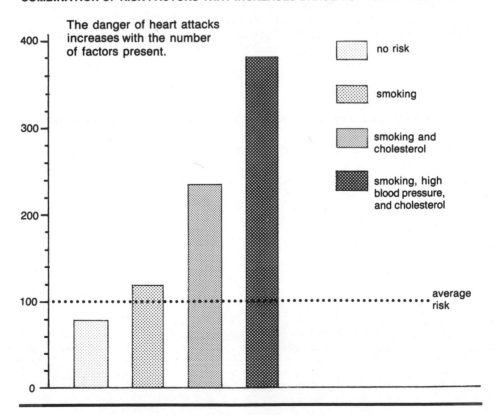

... will alter this grim picture. Specifics are indicated." Fortunately, once again, doctors now know a good deal more and can accomplish a good deal more. The tragedy involved in all these deaths is that something could be done about virtually every one of the risk factors.

To understand many of the recommendations currently being made for the prevention or treatment of atherosclerosis, and the interventions likely to be recommended in the near future, one must understand some of the insights gained during the past few years. Fortunately, what had seemed an unrelated series of observations and notions is now converging into a simplified story. Doctors and patients can look forward, therefore, to a much more rational and systematic use of the information to improve prevention and treatment.

Among the factors now recognized as contributing in the development of atherosclerotic plaque are lipoprotein cholesterol, damage to the endothelial cells lining the blood vessels, and adhesion of platelets to these damaged cells. It has become apparent that these are related phenomena.

## "GOOD" CHOLESTEROL AND "BAD" CHOLESTEROL

Although cholesterol has been recognized as a prime player for many years, scientists have recently learned a great deal about some of the details of cholesterol metabolism that has provided new insight and new approaches. Cholesterol does not circulate in free solution in the blood but rather travels attached to a protein, called a lipoprotein. There are a number of different lipoproteins; these can be separated on the basis of their

---

**WARNING**

It has been reported that four out of five middle-aged American men are at risk of dying prematurely of heart disease, due to elevated cholesterol levels. Dr. Jeremiah Stamler, a cardiologist from Northwestern University, reported, "I think the numbers speak rather clearly for themselves. The optimal cholesterol level is 180, and 80 percent of this population is over 180. They're all at risk."

physical or chemical properties. That separation turns out to be important. About 60 to 75 percent of total plasma cholesterol is transported, normally, in the form of a low-density lipoprotein, or LDL. A smaller percentage, perhaps 20 percent, is transported as a high-density lipoprotein, or HDL. LDL cholesterol is "bad" cholesterol, contributing to coronary artery disease in several ways. Conversely, HDL cholesterol is "good" cholesterol.

The protein that carries HDL removes cholesterol from its location in the arteries and returns it to the liver for disposition. Maneuvers known to reduce the likelihood of coronary artery disease, such as exercise and consuming a limited amount of alcohol daily, appear to work at least in part by increasing the amount of HDL relative to the total cholesterol. One or two ounces a day of hard whisky (or two three-ounce glasses of wine or one twelve-ounce bottle of beer) appears to be better than either total abstinence or consuming more from the point of view of developing coronary artery disease. Cigarette smoking and the progesteronelike hormones in the birth control pill reduce HDL. The more HDL cholesterol there is, the more that is being mobilized from various locations in the body and being removed. Some of the new drugs available for treating high cholesterol actually increase HDL cholesterol and thus help reduce the likelihood of artery disease.

It has long been recognized that some individuals inherit an abnormality in cholesterol metabolism that results in a striking acceleration of the atherosclerotic process. Serum cholesterol in these individuals is strikingly elevated, and severe coronary artery disease develops in the very young, even in the absence of associated risk factors. Severe heart disease is often present in teenagers, and many die before the age of twenty years.

Familial hypercholesterolemia has a dominant inheritance, so if one parent carries the gene, there will be an increase in serum cholesterol, some abnormalities in fundamental chemistry, and premature atherosclerosis. Although it is uncommon, with the frequency of about 1 in 500 in the population, a substantial number of the individuals who have a heart attack before the age of fifty in fact have this underlying problem. Even more rare, perhaps with a frequency of 1 in 1 million, is the devastating effect of both parents carrying this gene. In that case, the serum cholesterol level is very high from early years, fat accumulates in the skin, and coronary artery disease may express itself by the age of ten.

Brown and Goldstein, at Southwestern Medical School of the University of Texas, in Dallas, were awarded the Nobel Prize for dissecting the mechanism of this process in 1986. They showed that these individuals lack a receptor that normally removed low-density lipoprotein from the blood. The receptor is critical in controlling plasma LDL in humans.

Important insights involve the gene carrier. These individuals have less severe elevations of serum cholesterol but are nonetheless at higher risk for premature coronary artery disease. Although the homozygous form (the complete expression of the disease, inherited from both parents) is rare, the frequency of the gene in the population is sufficient that a substantial percentage of individuals with high serum cholesterol and a family history of disease, in fact, carry this trait. Now that scientists have identified the mechanism, and have means for identifying such patients, more specific treatment for them will be forthcoming.

The ratio of HDL to LDL is important. Most laboratories today present the total cholesterol—which is mostly made up of LDL cholesterol—and the HDL cholesterol. If the ratio of total cholesterol to HDL cholesterol is less than 4 to 1, the risk of developing heart problems is low. If it is greater than 6 to 1, the risk of developing heart problems is substantial. The intermediate area is a "gray zone" of risk.

## TREATMENT OF INCREASED SERUM CHOLESTEROL

Recent data from interventional studies have strengthened the cause-and-effect relationship between an increase in serum cholesterol and coronary artery disease. In 1984 and 1985, the reports from the Lipid Research Clinics Coronary Primary Prevention Trial were published. The patients had followed a prescribed diet and had used a lipid-lowering agent, cholestyramine. Overall, a 9 percent reduction in serum cholesterol was associated with a 19 percent reduction in mortality and heart attack rate, compared with patients who received no drug and had only dietary modification. In a subgroup of patients in whom cholesterol level was reduced by 25 percent, there was a more impressive 49 percent reduction in coronary heart disease mortality and heart attack rate. In 1987 the Helsinki Heart Study examined the effects of diet and the use of another drug, gemfibrozil, on coronary heart disease events in men with an

**KEEPING TRACK OF CHOLESTEROL LEVELS**

| Age | Moderate Risk (Top 25%) |
|-----|-------------------------|
| 20–29 | Over 200 mg/dl |
| 30–39 | Over 220 mg/dl |
| 40 + | Over 240 mg/dl |

| Age | High Risk (Top 10%) |
|-----|---------------------|
| 20–29 | Over 220 mg/dl |
| 30–39 | Over 240 mg/dl |
| 40 + | Over 260 mg/dl |

| Age | Goal |
|-----|------|
| 20–29 | Under 180 mg/dl |
| 30–39 | Under 200 mg/dl |
| 40 + | Under 200 mg/dl |

Source: Adapted from the NIH Consensus Development Conference, "Lowering Blood Cholesterol to Prevent Heart Disease," 1984

elevated serum cholesterol. In a group on drug treatment, a 9 percent reduction in LDL cholesterol, associated with a 10 percent increase in HDL cholesterol, resulted in a significant 34 percent reduction in coronary heart disease events. These studies have made it clear that correcting abnormal blood lipids can result in achievement of the desired goal—prevention of heart attacks.

Most experts still believe that the first approach in every person should involve a combination of diet and exercise. For those with a striking abnormality of serum cholesterol, the diet will generally be prescribed along with appropriate drugs from the onset of treatment. For those with milder abnormalities, diet and exercise will be employed first, and drugs only if the combination is ineffective.

Dietary treatment occurs in two stages. The least stringent diet calls for reducing dietary fat to less than 30 percent of the total calories. In the average U.S. diet, fat currently accounts for almost 40 percent of total calories. This diet also calls for less than 10 percent of total calories in the form of saturated fat and a reduction of cholesterol intake to less than 300 milligrams per day. Calorie restriction and an exercise program are recommended for those who are overweight, and walking is stressed as an important element in any exercise program.

If after three months the cholesterol goal has remained elusive, it is generally helpful to involve a registered dietician who will help decide whether a more stringent diet is required. The more stringent diet involves an intake of saturated fat representing less than 7 percent of calories and an intake of cholesterol to less than 200 milligrams per day.

A wide and growing range of drugs is available to supplement diet and exercise should the tougher diet also prove inadequate. Their selection depends in large part on the specific pattern of abnormal blood lipids that you have and with your ability to deal with the adverse effects of each of the agents. For an individual with an increase in LDL cholesterol alone, and for whom diet and exercise have been ineffective in reducing the cholesterol level satisfactorily, the most widely used drugs are cholestyramine and cholestipol. Both are resins that bind bile acids in the intestine and thus remove cholesterol from the body. They can reduce plasma LDL cholesterol by about 20 to 25 percent. These drugs are prescribed as powders that must be mixed with water or fruit juice. They are available in packets, for convenience, but are more economical when purchased in cans or bottles. They are usually taken in divided doses each day with meals. Some persons prefer one to the other, but either can cause gastrointestinal side effects including queasiness, nausea, bloating, and constipation. Many find them to be unpalatable, and others tolerate them well. If you are taking other drugs such as digitalis, a beta-blocker, or a thiazide diuretic, these drugs should be taken at least one hour before or four hours after one of these resins, since the resins interfere with absorption.

If these agents are not well tolerated, the next choice is niacin, which may be employed alone (to reduce plasma LDL cholesterol by about 20 percent) or combined with cholestyramine or colestipol, in which case plasma LDL cholesterol may be reduced over 40 percent. Niacin must be taken with meals because it can irritate the stomach, and for this reason it is never prescribed for someone who has a history of peptic ulcer. For those with gout or diabetes, niacin can be a problem, since it raises serum uric acid and can make diabetes worse. The most common complaint is flushing of the skin, which can be prominent and which may be associated with itchiness. Some approaches to dealing with this problem include the use of a single aspirin daily, with a gradual increase in the dose so that tolerance to the flushing can be developed.

In patients in whom the abnormality in blood lipids also includes an elevated triglyceride level, niacin is often chosen as the first agent. An alternative is the drug mentioned as part of the Helsinki Heart Study, gemfibrozil. It may cause muscle aches or muscle damage and is never used in the individual with kidney or liver disease. In persons with very high triglyceride levels, the use of fish oil capsules containing EPA can be very helpful. In the person with primarily an increase in LDL cholesterol, the effect of gemfibrozil tends to be limited— reducing LDL cholesterol by about 9 percent as described in the Helsinki Heart Study—but it clearly has an impact on the evolution of heart disease.

A new drug, lovastatin, has become available for the treatment of increased blood cholesterol when diet and exercise have been ineffective in achieving a goal serum cholesterol level. This agent works by blocking the enzyme that controls the production of cholesterol. Through a chain of reactions, it then lowers the concentration of LDL cholesterol and increases the HDL, or good, cholesterol. In a recent study, this agent reduced LDL levels by an average of 39 percent in 101 patients treated for eighteen weeks, substantially higher than the reduction achieved in the Lipid Research Clinics studies cited above. The agent also seems to be better tolerated than many predecessors. For comparison, even the most rigorous diets generally result in only a 5 to 15 percent drop in an individual's cholesterol, unless the patient's earlier pattern had involved the use of an enormous number of eggs and considerable quantities of marbled beef, liver, and cholesterol-rich dairy products.

## THE BLOOD VESSELS' DAMAGED LINING

LDL cholesterol also plays a role in endothelial damage. A single layer of very smooth cells, the endothelium, lines the inside of blood vessels. Atherosclerosis begins in the layer just below the endothelium, the intima. Endothelial injury, from whatever cause, results in easy access of materials, including LDL cholesterol, to the intimal area beyond the endothelial cells. High blood pressure can injure the endothelium. Cigarette smoking can injure the endothelium. This is how two of the known risk factors for atherosclerosis work. The third cause of endothelial cell injury is LDL cholesterol, per se. For reasons that are not entirely clear, exposure of endothelial cells to high concentrations of LDL cholesterol injures them, allowing the LDL to gain access to the intima, the place where atherosclerosis occurs. Thus, LDL cholesterol can help bring itself to the very place that we do not want it.

The endothelial cells prevent blood clotting from occurring. When the endothelial cells are disrupted, as occurs with a cut, this normal process limits the amount of bleeding that goes on. There are several important steps in this process. First, small cells that circulate in the blood, called platelets, are attracted to a disrupted area and stick there. Because they are normally sticky, and because the local tissue reaction to disrupted endothelium initiates a chemical process that makes them more sticky, the result is the formation of a plug. After that, the setting is created for the activation of certain proteins in the blood that lead to the formation of a blood clot that more permanently seals the disruption.

With endothelial cell injury, platelets collect, even though there is no hemorrhage to stop. This has several implications. First, the platelets tend to form a plug and thus reduce blood flow in the artery. Second, certain hormones that cause blood vessel spasm are released from the platelets. Among these, two, serotonin and thromboxane, are especially important. When platelets are activated, the release of thromboxane promotes further spasm and further platelet stickiness. (See figure 16.)

---

### SUCCESSES

The advances made in the last twenty years in understanding atherosclerosis have made a big difference. Between 1962 and 1982, the mortality rate from coronary heart disease dropped 37 percent. Based on the calculations of Dr. Lee Goldman and Dr. E. Francis Cook of Harvard Medical School, about 40 percent of the decline in mortality can be credited to medical interventions such as coronary care units, drug therapy, treatment of high blood pressure, improved resuscitation techniques, and coronary bypass surgery.

But two other improvements account for more than half the decline in the death rate—people have been cutting down on their consumption of cigarettes and fatty foods.

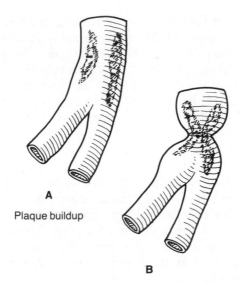

**A**

Plaque buildup

**B**

Spasm causing blockage

**Figure 16.   Partially Obstructed Artery**

Plaque buildup has caused some obstruction in the artery **(A)**. Spasm involving the artery wall around the plaque **(B)** can add to the obstruction. Specific treatments are available for spasm induced in this way.

## ASPIRIN AS A RISK REDUCER

Ordinary, common aspirin—so widely used for fever and pain that many do not think of it as a drug—in low concentrations blocks the formation of thromboxane. Indeed, a low dose of aspirin has been shown to reduce complications related to atherosclerosis in the patient at risk of a stroke, and perhaps of a heart attack. There is every reason to believe that the action of aspirin reflects its ability to reduce thromboxane formation when platelet aggregation occurs. This reduces the tendency to spasm and reduces platelet stickiness.

## FISH AS A RISK REDUCER

Part of the beneficial action enjoyed by those who eat fish, or use fish oil, is related to thromboxane production. Thrombox-

ane is derived from a fatty acid that comes from animal tissues. Fish oil contains a different fatty acid, called eicosapentaenoic acid (EPA), which results in the formation of a hormone that resembles thromboxane but lacks thromboxane's bad features. EPA works by thus "getting in the way" of thromboxane production. As a consequence, there is less tendency to platelet aggregation in individuals who eat a substantial amount of fish, and perhaps less spasm.

Investigators examining the origins of the atherosclerotic plaque also recognize additional factors. Proliferation of different cells within the plaque occurs, for example. Although none of the preventive measures or approaches to treatment have yet addressed that information, it seems likely that they will do so in the near future.

# 8

# Risk Factors for Atherosclerotic Disease—What to Do About Them

Since many of the factors in the development of atherosclerosis are known, various suggestions can be made concerning the reduction of risk.

## FAT

Serum cholesterol, especially LDL cholesterol, is clearly an important factor in the development of atherosclerotic disease. What can we do about it? A recent study shows that a large reduction in blood cholesterol can slow and sometimes even reverse fatty deposits that clog arteries. Many people, the data indicate, may be able to improve the health of their arteries.

Americans and others in industrialized society eat too much fat. About 40 to 50 percent of the calories in a typical diet consist of fat. The percentage is even higher for those who frequently eat "junk food," found in a fast-food restaurant. All experts agree that no more than about one-third of the calories should come in the form of fat, and some suggest that even less is appropriate.

### Polyunsaturated Fat Versus Saturated Fat

The nature of the fat eaten is important. Surely everyone has heard about polyunsaturated fats. Animal fat and butter are examples of fat made up of saturated fatty acids. The terms *saturated* and *unsaturated* come from chemical nomenclature. *Saturation* means "adding hydrogen." As a consequence of adding hydrogen (hydrogenation), the fat will tend to be solid at

**115**

A Washington-based consumer group, the Center for Science in the Public Interest, reports that the following fast-food chains fry their food in heavily hydrogenated oil or beef fat:

- Arby's
- Big Boy
- Burger King
- Hardee's
- McDonald's
- Popeyes
- Wendy's
- Howard Johnson's
- Church's
- Kentucky Fried Chicken

Dr. Howard Eder, recipient of the American Heart Association 1985 Distinguished Accomplishment Award, says that the moderately hydrogenated vegetable oil used by Denny's, Friendly's, and Papa Gino's is "acceptable."

room temperature. Unsaturated fatty acids tend to be liquid, an oil at room temperature. Eating saturated fat raises total cholesterol, especially LDL cholesterol. Eating unsaturated fat with the same number of calories will depress the levels of LDL cholesterol. By replacing saturated with polyunsaturated fats; prudently decreasing the intake of cholesterol-rich foods such as liver, marbled beef, and butter, cream, and other dairy products; and limiting egg yolks to three per week, one can reduce serum cholesterol by 10 to 15 percent.

**Vegetable Oils — Not All Alike**

There are some important caveats. One involves the use of "vegetable oils." Coconut oil, for example, has found wide and increasing use to replace dairy products, especially in nondairy creamers and pastry icings. Despite its vegetable origin, there is evidence from studies in animals that substitution of coconut oil for butterfat in fact makes atherosclerosis worse. Similarly, although peanut oil is in part unsaturated, it has been shown to be effective in inducing atherosclerosis in animals. Although this does not translate in a straightforward way to the impact of the use of small amounts of peanut oil in human beings, the influence of coconut and peanut oil does suggest that it is not enough to read a label for its vegetable oil content or even for how unsaturated the fat is. Prudent judgment suggests that we turn to sources that are believed to be more benign, such as polyunsaturated fats found in oils from safflowers, sunflowers, corn, and soybeans. Be careful, since some vegetable fat can be turned into saturated fat by hydrogenation. Check labels before you buy.

Monounsaturated fats seem to be more neutral and do not change cholesterol levels. In this category are olives and olive oil. Please be reminded, as mentioned above, that peanut oil, although monounsaturated, can predispose to atherosclerosis in animal models.

## The Fat Content of Foods

Fat content and caloric content are not necessarily parallel. For example, a slice of chocolate cake or a generous slice of apple pie will provide between 250 and 350 calories, but the percentage from fat is about 45 percent. On the other hand, a doughnut is 175 calories and is 60 to 65 percent fat; an ounce of salami or bologna, having 75 to 90 calories, is 70 to 75 percent fat.

### FATTY ACID COMPOSITION OF OILS AND FATS

| Source | Polyunsaturated (%) | Monounsaturated (%) | Saturated (%) | P/S Ratio |
|---|---|---|---|---|
| Beef fat | 2 | 44 | 54 | less than 0.1 |
| Butter | 4 | 37 | 59 | less than 0.1 |
| Chicken fat | 27 | 29 | 44 | 0.6 |
| Coconut oil | 2 | 6 | 92 | less than 0.1 |
| Corn oil | 60 | 26 | 14 | 4.3 |
| Egg yolk | 14 | 51 | 35 | 0.4 |
| Lard | 14 | 46 | 40 | 0.4 |
| Olive oil | 15 | 69 | 16 | 0.9 |
| Palm oil | 10 | 37 | 53 | 0.2 |
| Peanut oil | 35 | 45 | 20 | 1.8 |
| Safflower oil | 78 | 11 | 11 | 7.1 |
| Soybean oil | 58 | 27 | 15 | 3.9 |
| Sunflower oil | 70 | 18 | 12 | 5.8 |

---

### YOU CAN DO WORSE THAN SHRIMP

Shrimp lovers may find the table below discouraging. But remembering that one egg yolk alone contains more than 250 milligrams of cholesterol makes shrimp less forbidding. Even people trying to control their blood cholesterol levels can sometimes indulge in shrimp. As for lobster and crab, their bad reputation as foods rich in cholesterol is undeserved.

| Source | Milligrams cholesterol per 4 ounces |
|---|---|
| Shrimp | 181 |
| Crab | 113 |
| Lobster | 94 |
| Chicken (light meat) | 91 |
| Fish (lean) | 74 |

---

Eat a typical quarter-pound hamburger, french fries, and a milk shake and you will ingest an artery-clogging fifteen to twenty teaspoons of fat—more than the ten teaspoons or so that a person should consume in an entire day. We all know that chicken and fish are healthier than beef, but if you get them at your local fast-food emporium, the filet of fish sandwich or small order of fried chicken nuggets may have *twice* as much fat as a regular hamburger because of the way it is prepared.

To compound the problem, many fast-food chains fry their food in pure beef fat rather than in liquid vegetable oil. They know we have come to love that flavor. Not only are the fried chicken, fish, and potatoes layered with fat, but also the fat is highly saturated. It is just plain unhealthy.

Does this mean absolute denial? No. When a trip to a fast-food restaurant seems the best solution to obtaining a quick and inexpensive meal, choose pizza rather than a traditional hamburger. It is high in carbohydrates and, especially if topped with tomato sauce and vegetables and without extra cheese, is a nutritious meal. Even with extra cheese, pizza has marginal fat and cholesterol compared with the alternatives. Chili has a high sodium content but is a better choice than hamburger, since you get a substantial amount of kidney beans with the ground beef, and thus substantial fiber with less animal fat.

Order small portions and avoid the sauces and salad dressings. Many places now provide low-calorie dressings as an alternative.

## Fish Oil

Several decades ago, it occurred to a number of individuals that the diet eaten by Eskimos presented a puzzle. Like many people from nonindustrialized areas, this group has a much lower frequency of heart attacks than does a population from an industrialized area. But unlike the majority of nonindustrialized groups, its diet contains as much fat or more as a European or typical U.S. diet. Cardiovascular disease is also much lower in an Okinawan population that shares with the Eskimos a high intake of fat and fish. Interestingly, their serum cholesterol average is not different from that of the inhabitants of mainland Japan.

These observations focused attention on the potential utility of fish oils in place of animal sources of fat. A very important epidemiological study, performed in Holland (see chapter 1) provided the most compelling evidence for the fact that replacing animal fat with fish oils is a good strategy. It should be obvious that having more fish in one's diet is very different

**EPA CONTENTS OF FISH**

| Species | Omega-3 content (approximate grams per 3½ ounces) | Species | Omega-3 content (approximate grams per 3½ ounces) |
|---|---|---|---|
| Sardines, Norway | 5.1 | Rainbow trout | 0.5 |
| Mackerel, Atlantic | 2.5 | King crab | 0.5 |
| Tuna, bluefin | 1.6 | Mussels | 0.5 |
| Herring, Atlantic | 1.6 | Lobster, shrimp | 0.3–0.4 |
| Sablefish | 1.4 | Scallops | 0.3 |
| Salmon, chinook | 1.4 | Cod, flounder | 0.3 |
| Salmon, sockeye | 1.2 | | |
| Salmon, pink | 1.0 | *For comparison:* | |
| Bluefish | 1.2 | | |
| Whiting | 0.8 | Chicken breast, skinless | .03 |
| Pollock | 0.5 | Ground beef | trace |

Source: *USDA Handbook No. 8; Journal of the American Dietetic Association,* June 1986.

from supplementing our already high-fat diets with fish oil. It is also not clear that fish was effective only because of the content of eicosapentaenoic acid. The authors of the Dutch study were careful to point out that the eicosapentaenoic acid content of the amount of fish consumed was likely to be 400 milligrams a day or less, very much less than the supplement generally recommended (see page 13).

What shall one do with this information? The prudent answer is to replace two traditional meals each week with fish, ideally broiled or prepared in ways that will not increase the fat content. That falls far short of the Eskimo-level doses of eicosapentaenoic acid, estimated to be 10 grams per day, the basis for suggestions about supplementation.

When it comes to the marketplace, discussion of nutrition resembles discussion of religion, politics, and sex. The subject is emotional, the real product is often intangible, and the profits can be substantial. The debate over the utility and merit of supplements is at present not resolvable. A prudent reaction suggests a reduction in total fat, a reduction in saturated fat and replacement with fat from polyunsaturated sources, and two fish meals a week. It seems unlikely that one can have one's cake and eat it too. There is no evidence that taking fish oils as a supplement—without readjusting one's diet and lifestyle—will significantly reduce cholesterol levels.

### RELATIONSHIP OF SERUM CHOLESTEROL TO THE CORONARY DEATH RATE

| Serum Cholesterol Level (milligrams/100 deciliters blood) | Coronary Death Rate (age adjusted) |
|---|---|
| 140–159 | 0.8% |
| 160–179 | 2.1 |
| 180–199 | 2.1 |
| 200–219 | 2.5 |
| 220–239 | 3.1 |
| 240–259 | 3.6 |
| 260–279 | 3.1 |
| 280–299 | 6.4 |
| 300–319 | 7.2 |
| greater than 320 | 14.4 |

## CHOLESTEROL CONTENT OF FOODS

| Food | Amount | Cholesterol (milligrams) |
|---|---|---|
| Liver | 3 oz. | 372 |
| Egg | 1 | 252 |
| Ladyfingers | 4 | 157 |
| Custard | 1/2 cup | 139 |
| Sardines | 3-1/4 oz. | 129 |
| Apple or custard pie | 1/8 of 9″ pie | 120 |
| Waffles—mix, egg, milk | 1 (9″ × 9″) | 112 |
| Lemon meringue pie | 1/8 of 9″ pie | 98 |
| Veal | 3 oz. | 86 |
| Turkey, dark meat, no skin | 3 oz. | 86 |
| Lamb | 3 oz. | 83 |
| Beef | 3 oz. | 80 |
| Pork | 3 oz. | 76 |
| Spaghetti and meatballs | 1 cup | 75 |
| Lobster | 3 oz. | 72 |
| Turkey, light meat, no skin | 3 oz. | 65 |
| Chicken breast | 1/2 breast | 63 |
| Noodles, whole egg | 1 cup, cooked | 50 |
| Clams | 1/2 cup | 50 |
| Macaroni and cheese | 1 cup | 42 |
| Chicken, drumstick | 1 | 39 |
| Oysters | 3 oz. | 38 |
| Fish fillet | 3 oz. | 34–75 |
| Whole milk | 8 oz. | 34 |
| Salmon, canned | 3 oz. | 30 |
| Hot dog | 1 | 27 |
| Cheddar or Swiss cheese | 1 oz. | 28 |
| Rice pudding with raisins | 1 cup | 29 |
| Ice cream | 1/2 cup | 27–49 |
| American processed cheese | 1 oz. | 25 |
| Low-fat milk (2%) | 8 oz. | 22 |
| Heavy whipping cream | 1 tbs. | 20 |
| Mozzarella, part skim | 1 oz. | 18 |
| Brownies | 1 (1-3/4″ × 1-3/4″ × 1-1/8″) | 17 |
| Yogurt, plain | 8 oz. | 17 |
| Cream cheese | 1 tbs. | 16 |
| Cottage cheese | 1/2 cup | 12–24 |
| Butter | 1 pat/tsp. | 12 |
| Mayonnaise | 1 tbs. | 10 |
| Sour cream | 1 tbs. | 8 |
| Half-and-half | 1 tbs. | 6 |
| Cottage cheese, dry curd | 1/2 cup | 6 |
| Nonfat milk/buttermilk | 8 oz. | 5 |
| Margarine | | 0 |
| Beans, grains, nuts, fruits, vegetables | | 0 |

### PERCENTAGE OF FAT CALORIES IN SELECTED FOODS

| Food | Amount | Fat Calories | Total Calories | Percent Fat |
|------|--------|--------------|----------------|-------------|
| **Beverages** | | | | |
| Beer, wine | 1 serving | 0 | 85–150 | 0 |
| Coffee, tea | 1 serving | 0 | 0 | 0 |
| Fruit juice | 6 oz. | 0 | 75–110 | 0 |
| **Dairy Products** | | | | |
| Milk chocolate, cocoa mix | 1 cup | 108 | 245 | 44 |
| Milk | | | | |
| whole | 1 cup | 81 | 160 | 50 |
| 2% | 1 cup | 45 | 145 | 31 |
| nonfat | 1 cup | trace | 90 | less than 1 |
| buttermilk | 1 cup | trace | 90 | less than 1 |
| Cheese | | | | |
| cheddar | 1 oz. | 81 | 115 | 70 |
| cottage, creamed | 1 cup | 90 | 260 | 35 |
| cottage, uncreamed | 1 cup | 9 | 170 | 5.3 |
| cream | 1 cu. in. | 54 | 60 | 90 |
| parmesan | 1 oz. | 81 | 130 | 2 |
| Swiss | 1 oz. | 72 | 105 | 69 |
| processed | 1 oz. | 81 | 105 | 77 |
| cheese food | 1 tbs. | 27 | 45 | 60 |
| Cream | | | | |
| half-and-half | 1 cup | 252 | 325 | 78 |
| sour | 1 cup | 423 | 485 | 87 |
| whipping, light | 1 cup | 675 | 715 | 94 |
| whipping, heavy | 1 cup | 810 | 840 | 96 |
| Imitation creamers | | | | |
| powdered | 1 tsp. | 9 | 10 | 90 |
| liquid | 1 tbs. | 18 | 20 | 90 |
| Custard | 1 cup | 135 | 305 | 44 |
| Ice cream | 1 cup | 126 | 255 | 49 |
| Ice milk | 1 cup | 63 | 200 | 31 |
| Yogurt | | | | |
| low fat | 1 cup | 36 | 125 | 29 |
| whole fat | 1 cup | 72 | 150 | 49 |
| **Meat, Poultry, Fish, Shellfish; Related Products** | | | | |
| Bacon | 2 slices | 72 | 90 | 80 |
| Beef | | | | |
| hamburger | | | | |
| regular | 3 oz. | 153 | 245 | 63 |
| lean | 3 oz. | 90 | 185 | 49 |
| steak, broiled | | | | |
| lean only | 2 oz. | 36 | 115 | 31 |
| lean and fat | 3 oz. | 243 | 330 | 74 |

### PERCENTAGE OF FAT CALORIES IN SELECTED FOODS (continued)

| Food | Amount | Fat Calories | Total Calories | Percent Fat |
|---|---|---|---|---|
| roast, oven-cooked rib | | | | |
| lean only | 1.8 oz. | 63 | 125 | 50 |
| lean and fat | 3 oz. | 306 | 375 | 81 |
| roast, oven-cooked heel of round | | | | |
| lean only | 2.7 oz. | 27 | 125 | 22 |
| lean and fat | 3 oz. | 63 | 165 | 38 |
| canned, corned | 3 oz. | 90 | 185 | 49 |
| Chicken | | | | |
| flesh only (broiled) | 3 oz. | 27 | 115 | 23 |
| drumstick (fried) | 2.1 oz. | 36 | 90 | 40 |
| Chili con carne | | | | |
| with beans | 1 cup | 135 | 335 | 40 |
| without beans | 1 cup | 342 | 510 | 67 |
| Pork | | | | |
| ham | | | | |
| light cured | 3 oz. | 171 | 245 | 70 |
| luncheon | 2 oz. | 90 | 135 | 67 |
| roast | 3 oz. | 216 | 310 | 70 |
| sausage | 1 oz. | 63 | 90 | 70 |
| bologna | 2 slices | 63 | 80 | 79 |
| Fish | | | | |
| clams | 3 oz. | 9 | 45 | 20 |
| crab meat | 3 oz. | 18 | 85 | 21 |
| oysters | 1 cup | 36 | 160 | 23 |
| salmon | 3 oz. | 45 | 120 | 38 |
| shrimp | 3 oz. | 9 | 100 | 9 |
| tuna, canned in oil | 3 oz. | 63 | 170 | 37 |
| **Beans, Peas, Nuts** | | | | |
| Almonds | 1 cup | 693 | 850 | 82 |
| Beans | | | | |
| great northern | 1 cup | 9 | 210 | 4 |
| navy | 1 cup | 9 | 225 | 4 |
| Cashews | 1 cup | 576 | 785 | 73 |
| Peanuts | 1 cup | 648 | 840 | 77 |
| Peas, split | 1 cup | 9 | 290 | 3 |
| **Vegetables** | | | | |
| Asparagus through zucchini | | trace | | less than 1 |
| Exceptions: | | | | |
| Candied sweet potatoes | 1 | 63 | 295 | 21 |
| All fried, sauteed, or buttered vegetables | | | | |

## FIBER

What could be more attractive than the notion that eating foods that contain a substantial amount of fiber—that is, the parts of plant foods that are generally not digestible by humans and so provide more bulk—would be healthy? The range of claims made for fiber is substantial, and the advertising of breakfast food cereals has provided continuing reinforcement.

The inclusion of whole grain breads and cereals, fruits and vegetables, and dried beans and peas in the diet is not a bad idea. Such foods certainly help in weight-reducing diets by substituting bulky, satisfying foods for those that have large amounts of fats and sugars. There is evidence that the change in bowel habit so induced will change the pressure in the colon and thus reduce the likelihood of the development of fingerlike pouches, called diverticula, which can become inflamed. That is reasonable and supported by substantial evidence. Most of the suggestions about cancer prevention, however, are still poorly supported.

Somewhere on middle ground is the likelihood that fiber will help with diet and the control of caloric intake and perhaps even affect blood lipids. The risk of making increased fiber intake an important part of one's lifestyle change is the feeling that one has accomplished a great deal. Chances are the accomplishment is not that great.

## ALCOHOLIC BEVERAGES

There has been long-standing interest in the relation of alcohol intake to cardiovascular disease. Alchohol abuse is certainly unhealthy for the liver, and sustained heavy alcohol use makes any kind of calorie control impossible. Alcohol provides 7 calories per gram, so an ounce provides over 200 calories. For comparison, sugar provides only 4 calories per gram. For some individuals with elevated blood lipids, excess intake of alcohol aggravates the condition. Excessive alcohol intake has also been reported to be associated with at least some increase in blood pressure.

There is, however, some evidence from epidemiological studies to suggest a preventive effect of moderate daily intake of alcoholic beverages. One or two ounces of hard liquor, or its equivalent in wine (about six ounces) or beer (about twelve ounces), taken daily has reduced the likelihood of a heart attack in two reasonably well controlled studies.

There is even a suggestion as to the mechanism: alcohol in those doses seems to increase the level of high-density lipoprotein cholesterol, the "good" cholesterol, though this is controversial.

## COFFEE

The caffeine in coffee can induce distinct cardiovascular changes including an increase in heart rate and some (generally benign) heart irregularities. Evidence for caffeine as a risk factor for coronary artery disease has been mixed. In late 1986, an important study from Johns Hopkins University in Baltimore described an experience with 1,000 white male physicians who had been studied for an average of twenty-five years. This is obviously a very substantial study. Individuals who drank five or more cups of coffee a day had 2.8 times as many episodes involving their heart as did those who drank none. Those who drank an intermediate amount, three or four cups per day, had twice as many. Although heavy coffee drinkers were more likely to be heavy smokers and to have somewhat higher cholesterol levels than those who drank no coffee, the association of coronary disease to coffee was sustained even when these factors were accounted for by statistical techniques. This report adds credibility to the long-standing notion that coffee might be a hazard. Again, for those at risk, the information suggests that it would be wise to limit coffee drinking, though by no means is it necessary to discontinue its use.

## OVERWEIGHT — HOW SERIOUS A PROBLEM?

Being overweight (see the table on pages 126–127) has long been recognized as making people more vulnerable to atherosclerosis and coronary artery disease. It is not clear whether overweight itself — apart from the impact of overeating and too little exercise on blood cholesterol, high blood pressure, and the tendency to diabetes — has its own aggravating effect. Nevertheless, exercise is good for you; it is necessary to control calories if you want to deal with the problem of blood lipids, which are clearly an important contributor to atherosclerotic disease; and

## HOW MUCH WEIGHT IS "OVERWEIGHT"?

Since 1983, when the Metropolitan Life Insurance Company updated its tables of desirable weights, there has been controversy about how much weight is "overweight." Below is a table showing contrasting versions of healthy weights. Using the same data used by Metropolitan Life, the Gerontology Research Center of the National Institute on Aging concluded that approved weights for those in their fifties and sixties ought to be more lenient.

On the other hand, the American Heart Association disapproves of even the lower weights quoted by Metropolitan Life, finding them *too* lenient.

### METROPOLITAN LIFE

| Height | Women | | | Men | | |
|--------|---------------|----------------|----------------|---------------|----------------|----------------|
|        | Small Frame | Medium Frame | Large Frame | Small Frame | Medium Frame | Large Frame |
| 4'9" | 99–108 | 106–118 | 115–128 | | | |
| 4'10" | 100–110 | 108–120 | 117–131 | | | |
| 4'11" | 101–112 | 110–123 | 119–134 | | | |
| 5'0" | 103–115 | 112–126 | 122–137 | | | |
| 5'1" | 105–118 | 115–129 | 125–140 | 123–129 | 126–136 | 133–145 |
| 5'2" | 108–121 | 118–132 | 128–144 | 125–131 | 128–138 | 135–148 |
| 5'3" | 111–124 | 121–135 | 131–148 | 127–133 | 130–140 | 137–151 |
| 5'4" | 114–127 | 124–138 | 134–152 | 129–135 | 132–143 | 139–155 |
| 5'5" | 117–130 | 127–141 | 137–156 | 131–137 | 134–146 | 141–159 |
| 5'6" | 120–133 | 130–144 | 140–160 | 133–140 | 137–149 | 144–163 |
| 5'7" | 123–136 | 133–147 | 143–164 | 135–143 | 140–152 | 147–167 |
| 5'8" | 126–139 | 136–150 | 146–167 | 137–146 | 143–155 | 150–171 |
| 5'9" | 129–142 | 139–153 | 149–170 | 139–149 | 146–158 | 153–175 |
| 5'10" | 132–145 | 142–156 | 152–173 | 141–152 | 149–161 | 156–179 |
| 5'11" | | | | 144–155 | 152–165 | 159–183 |
| 6'0" | | | | 147–159 | 155–169 | 163–187 |
| 6'1" | | | | 150–163 | 159–173 | 167–192 |
| 6'2" | | | | 153–167 | 162–177 | 171–197 |
| 6'3" | | | | 157–171 | 166–182 | 176–202 |
| 6'4" | | | | | | |

All heights without shoes, weights in pounds without clothes.

GERONTOLOGY RESEARCH CENTER

| Height | Men and Women | | | | |
|---|---|---|---|---|---|
| | Ages 20–29 | Ages 30–39 | Ages 40–49 | Ages 50–59 | Ages 60–69 |
| 4'9" | | | | | |
| 4'10" | 84–111 | 92–119 | 99–127 | 107–135 | 115–142 |
| 4'11" | 87–115 | 95–123 | 103–131 | 111–139 | 119–147 |
| 5'0" | 90–119 | 98–127 | 106–135 | 114–143 | 123–152 |
| 5'1" | 93–123 | 101–131 | 110–140 | 118–148 | 127–157 |
| 5'2" | 96–127 | 105–136 | 113–144 | 122–153 | 131–163 |
| 5'3" | 99–131 | 108–140 | 117–149 | 126–158 | 135–168 |
| 5'4" | 102–135 | 112–145 | 121–154 | 130–163 | 140–173 |
| 5'5" | 106–140 | 115–149 | 125–159 | 134–168 | 144–179 |
| 5'6" | 109–144 | 119–154 | 129–164 | 138–174 | 148–184 |
| 5'7" | 112–148 | 122–159 | 133–169 | 143–179 | 153–190 |
| 5'8" | 116–153 | 126–163 | 137–174 | 147–184 | 158–196 |
| 5'9" | 119–157 | 130–168 | 141–179 | 151–190 | 162–201 |
| 5'10" | 122–162 | 134–173 | 145–184 | 156–195 | 167–207 |
| 5'11" | 126–167 | 137–178 | 149–190 | 160–201 | 172–213 |
| 6'0" | 129–171 | 141–183 | 153–195 | 165–207 | 177–219 |
| 6'1" | 133–176 | 145–188 | 157–200 | 169–213 | 182–225 |
| 6'2" | 137–181 | 149–194 | 162–206 | 174–219 | 187–232 |
| 6'3" | 141–186 | 153–199 | 166–212 | 179–225 | 192–238 |
| 6'4" | 144–191 | 157–205 | 171–218 | 184–231 | 197–244 |

**COOKING TIPS**

- Before cooking meat, make sure you have first trimmed off all the visible fat.

- Don't baste meat in its own drippings. Instead, try wine or some other prepared sauce.

- Steaming, baking, broiling, and braising are all healthier than frying. If you are roasting meat, try to keep the temperature low (350° F) to avoid sealing in fat.

- Mash potatoes with skim milk. As a general rule, substitute skim milk for whole milk.

- If a recipe calls for eggs, use the whites and throw the yolks away. This works for pancakes, cookies, and cakes. It will help you cut consumption of egg yolks to three per week.

- Choose lean cuts of beef. Make sure ground beef is "extra lean." Hot dogs, sausages, bacon, and luncheon meats are, unfortunately, usually high in cholesterol and saturated fat.

the treatment of high blood pressure and of diabetes mellitus is much more difficult in the overweight. Indeed, for both maturity onset diabetes and hypertension, the most straightforward, effective treatment is weight loss.

## HORMONES

Perhaps the most widely recognized fact is that women before the menopause are much less likely to have a heart attack than are men, matched for age. After the menopause, the difference shrinks. Women in their forties and early fifties who have undergone menopause have been found to have a threefold increase in the frequency of coronary artery events, compared with women of the same age who are still menstruating. The evidence on whether estrogen reversed that tendency is still unclear, as much of the evidence is conflicting.

Part of the confusion has come from investigators' pooling of the results from spontaneous menopause, which occurs very gradually, and surgical menopause. Surgical removal of the ovaries during a hysterectomy is a very common operation in this country. Treatment with estrogen in a dose just required to prevent disturbing menopausal symptoms reduced sharply the frequency of coronary artery events in women following surgical menopause but did nothing to coronary events in those in whom menopause occurred spontaneously. This study analyzing information obtained from more than 100,000 nurses who entered the study provides some clear indications as to when estrogen use is likely to be important. Estrogen use might be justifiable for a host of reasons, but its influence on coronary events appears to be restricted largely to those in whom menopause occurs abruptly following surgery.

Estrogen use in men, and perhaps in younger women, appears to be associated with an increase in the frequency of coronary artery disease.

A related question involves the effect of vasectomy. Studies in animal models showed more severe atherosclerotic disease after vasectomy, an effect that was unrelated to plasma lipid levels. Studies in vasectomized men, however, have not shown any evidence of an increased risk of atherosclerotic disease.

## EXERCISE

A gradual accumulation of evidence suggests that physical activity reduces the likelihood of atherosclerotic disease, especially coronary artery disease, though controversy continues. The obvious problem is the fact that individuals who choose to be physically active, either at work or in their leisure time, may differ in substantial ways from people who choose not to. Moreover, the assessment over the long term of how physically active someone has been is not straightforward. However, the bulk of available evidence indicates that physical activity does indeed help.

Perhaps the most persuasive studies were published recently by Dr. Ralph Paffenbarger and his associates at Stanford University. They have performed a careful, long-term evaluation of graduates of Harvard College who were assessed during their college years and for many years thereafter. These studies showed that individuals who maintain a high level of physical activity showed a sharp reduction in the number of coronary events. Fatal heart disease was seen to be almost twice as frequent among the least active people as it was among the most active. Not only that, these studies provided some quantitative information on how much exercise is actually required.

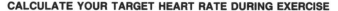

**CALCULATE YOUR TARGET HEART RATE DURING EXERCISE**

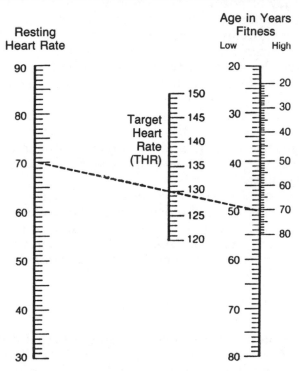

The target heart rate is the number of beats per minute your heart must have during exercise to increase the level of your cardiovascular fitness.

To calculate your target heart rate, do the following:

1. Find your *resting* heart rate. Sit down, relax, and count the number of times your pulse beats in one minute. This number is your resting heart rate. Make a mark on the chart above next to the appropriate number in the first column.

2. Ask yourself whether your fitness level is low or high. Then mark the chart appropriately for your age and fitness level. Notice that age is combined with level of fitness to decide where you fit on the spectrum. A fit person of sixty is at the same level, on this chart, as a person of forty-five who has just decided to get in shape.

3. Now draw a straight line between your resting heart rate and your point on the age/fitness spectrum. This line will intersect the target heart rate line— and there you have your target heart rate.

Identifying your target heart rate has a useful purpose. How do you decide whether you are achieving optimal cardiovascular benefit from your brisk walk or other form of exercise? The goal is to achieve your target heart rate. As you continue to exercise, and move from a low to a high fitness level, your target heart rate will change. Once again, this chart can be used to identify the new target heart rate.

The amount of exercise—the energy cost—required to provide measurable protection was 2,300 calories per week.

A three-mile walk in forty-five to sixty minutes has an energy cost of about 300 calories. Climbing a flight of stairs has an energy cost of about 10 calories. Thus, a daily brisk walk, lasting about forty-five minutes to an hour, and some stair climbing during the week will provide the level of brisk exercise required to achieve the goal of risk reduction. Moreover, burning that amount of additional energy every week represents about 10,000 calories a month, equivalent to a three-pound weight loss, without any change in food intake.

There is still disagreement as to whether a moderate amount of exercise not creating cardiovascular demands will improve risk. Ideally, exercise should raise one's heart rate to about two-thirds of the maximum. (See page 130 for information on how to calculate a "target heart rate" during exercise.)

## BLOOD PRESSURE

There is no doubt that an increase in blood pressure makes one susceptible to coronary artery disease and atherosclerotic disease elsewhere in the body. There is also no doubt that the higher the pressure, the greater the level of risk. What remains in doubt is which form of treatment for high blood pressure provides the optimal reduction in the likelihood of a heart attack or the development of peripheral arterial disease. The treatment of hypertension, however it is undertaken, clearly reduces the likelihood of a stroke.

The other message that has become clear is that the impact of high blood pressure on the likelihood of having coronary artery disease or atherosclerotic disease elsewhere interacts strongly with other risk factors. Thus, for example, the combination of high blood cholesterol, high blood pressure, and cigarette abuse produces a likelihood of heart attack that is substantially greater than the sum of the individual factors. To modify that course, it seems likely that effective treatment for all aspects must be undertaken.

## CIGARETTE SMOKING

The risk of a heart attack in cigarette-smoking men is about 60 percent higher than in nonsmoking men. The more one

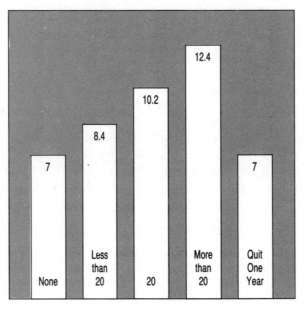

**CARDIOVASCULAR MORTALITY**
**(Average annual incidence per 1,000)**

Cigarettes smoked per day

smokes, the greater the risk. For those who smoke more than twenty cigarettes a day, the risk is doubled.

There is more bad news in recent studies. Reducing cigarette use to five per day in a heavy smoker does not change the nicotine load because the pattern of smoking changes so that each cigarette provides much more. Each cigarette was smoked down to the shortest possible level, and each inhalation of cigarette smoke was very deep. As a consequence, the total amount of nicotine absorbed was unchanged. The same caveat is involved in the attempt to switch to filter cigarettes.

However, complete cessation of cigarette smoking results in a extraordinarily rapid reversal in the increased risk of coronary artery disease. Within one year, the increased risk is gone.

## DIABETES MELLITUS

Diabetes can contribute to coronary artery disease in a number of ways. Whatever the contribution, diabetes merits treatment in its own right. For the individual who already is at high risk because of other risk factors, the urgency of following the treatment pattern established for the diabetes is clearly increased in importance.

## PERSONALITY PROFILE

Surely everyone has heard about "Type A behavior" as a contributor to coronary artery disease. The Type A personality is constantly trying to achieve more, and do more, and to do it in less and less time. Such individuals are characteristically portrayed as being aggressive, ambitious, and competitive. They are preoccupied with work and deadlines, often creating deadlines to increase their productivity. Urban society rewards Type A behavior, bringing out the tendency for people to push themselves.

What can we do about it? First, we can recognize that the evidence is controversial and mixed. Indeed, there is greater risk in being unsuccessful and uneducated. To the extent that the available evidence suggests that the time urgency experienced by the Type A personality might contribute to disease, it makes sense to create a personal environment in which times are set aside to relax. Interests that are scheduled as part of every week, unrelated to work or deadlines, are healthy. If they also provide a solution to the problem of a sedentary life, that is all to the good.

---

Do you
- finish other people's sentences?
- set self-imposed deadlines?
- walk and eat faster than those around you?
- become impatient when waiting for someone slower than you?

If so, take it with a grain of salt. The evidence about Type A personality as a risk factor is not conclusive.

# 9

# Angina Pectoris

There is a law of supply and demand applied to the heart. *Coronary insufficiency* is a generic term used to describe any abnormality of the coronary arteries sufficient to limit the supply of blood to the heart. The terms *ischemic heart disease, coronary artery disease, coronary heart disease*, and *atherosclerotic heart disease* are synonymous, implying some obstruction of the arteries that limits the blood supply. (The term *ischemic* is Greek for "too little blood.") The term *infarction*, as in *myocardial infarction*, indicates that some of the heart muscle has died, or undergone necrosis, as a result of insufficient blood supply. Pain in the chest that is related to a limitation of the blood supply to the heart—limited in relation to the heart's need—is known as angina pectoris. The blood supply, and the oxygen provided with it, may be adequate to cover the heart's requirements when the individual is at rest but becomes inadequate during the increased demands that occur, for example, with physical exertion, emotional stress, or a heavy meal. In the vast majority of cases, some obstruction to the coronary arteries, which supply blood to the heart, is present.

When the limitation of blood supply is temporary, brought on by exercise or some emotional state, the heart muscle is generally left intact. When the demand is more prolonged and the supply more severely limited, as occurs when the coronary artery disease is complicated by the development of a blood clot that blocks the coronary artery, the result is myocardial infarction—also called coronary thrombosis, or, in lay language, a heart attack.

The most common cause of angina pectoris is atherosclerosis involving the coronary arteries. At one time, syphilis involving the large artery that carries blood away from the heart,

| | |
|---|---|
| **ischemic heart disease** | synonyms for inadequate blood supply |
| **coronary artery disease** | to the heart, commonly caused by |
| **coronary heart disease** | atherosclerosis |
| **atherosclerotic heart disease** | |

**atherosclerosis:** a disease commonly aggravated by high LDL cholesterol levels, high blood pressure, or smoking, in which damage is done to the arteries by
- buildup of cholesterol,
- damage to the blood vessel lining, and/or
- clotting of increasingly "sticky" blood platelets.

**angina pectoris:** the "strangling" pain associated with ischemic heart disease, most commonly occurring when exercise or stress places demands on blood flow to the heart that damaged arteries cannot supply.

| | |
|---|---|
| **myocardial infarction** | synonyms for the death of part of the |
| **coronary thrombosis** | heart muscle, often caused by ischemic |
| **heart attack** | heart disease aggravated by a blood clot |
| | that clogs the coronary artery |

the aorta, was a relatively common cause, as were abnormalities of the aortic valve caused by rheumatic fever. These have now become distinctly uncommon. The factors involved in the development of atherosclerosis involving the coronary artery are those reviewed in chapters 7 and 8. If an individual has anemia, has a hyperactive thyroid gland, is very obese, carries a low blood-oxygen content because of lung disease or a congenital heart disease, the effort required to induce anginal pain is likely to be reduced.

High blood pressure is often associated with angina pectoris, through several mechanisms. First, for reasons reviewed earlier, high blood pressure tends to increase the likelihood of coronary artery disease. Second, high blood pressure increases the work required of the heart to keep blood circulating.

## VULNERABILITY TO ANGINA

At least 90 percent of individuals with angina pectoris are past the age of forty, and more than 70 percent are over fifty. When angina pectoris occurs in the younger person, there is usually a specific explanation such as the inheritance of an abnormality of blood lipids, a congenital abnormality of the coronary blood supply, or one of the factors described above that bring on angina. Men are involved much more frequently than women until women are well beyond the menopause.

As a result of the limited blood supply, there is a disproportion between the metabolic requirements of the heart muscle and the delivery of oxygen to satisfy those requirements. When supply is limited by the arterial disease, an increase in demand that occurs with exercise, emotion, sexual activity, or a heavy meal creates a setting in which the increased demand cannot be met by the supply. The result is abnormal metabolism in the heart and the stress signal of chest pain. The better the arteries, the more increase in demand is required before the supply becomes inadequate.

## CHARACTERISTICS OF THE PAIN

The term *angina pectoris* is unusual, having been used by an English physician over two hundred years ago to differentiate this form of chest pain from multiple other forms. He used the word *angina* to indicate a strangling quality as a distinctive feature of the chest pain. It is not really a disease but rather a syndrome characterized by sudden attacks of a distinctive pain that is usually in the chest behind the breastbone and commonly radiates to adjacent areas along the left upper arm to the jaw or to the back (see figure 17). The distinctive pain is often precipitated by physical effort, emotion, or a meal and is rapidly relieved by rest or by nitroglycerin. Pain that is localized on the left side of the chest below the nipple and overlies the heart directly is rarely due to angina pectoris, and pain that is described as sharp virtually never is due to it.

The pain of angina pectoris may be mild or severe, but whatever its intensity, it has a special quality that has been described variously as "constricting," "pressing," "boring," or "expanding." Some describe it as a sense of a band or vice around the chest or as a feeling of tightness, rather than a sharp or knifelike discomfort; it is constant and not throbbing. Still others describe it not as a pain but rather as a sense of oppression or choking.

Occasionally, the sensation of strangling or choking may be felt as respiratory difficulty, but the feeling differs from the shortness of breath that occurs in other problems involving the lungs or in heart failure.

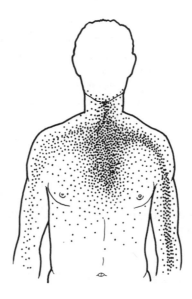

**Figure 17.   Areas of Anginal Pain**

The shaded area represents the distribution of the pain of angina pectoris. The darkest areas—involving the center of the chest, the lower neck, and the left arm—are the most typical areas where the pain occurs. On occasion, the pain can be distributed in the jaw, along the right arm, or in the upper abdomen.

The pain often has an insistent quality that compels the person experiencing it to remain as quiet as possible and, if the person has been running, walking, or in any way exerting himself or herself to stop the activity.

Certain psychic features often are found to accompany the pain, and the fear of immediate or impending death that sometimes occurs was recognized by the British physician who named the process over two centuries ago. In fact, death during a typical anginal attack is distinctly uncommon despite the origin of the attack in the heart.

An attack of angina pectoris usually lasts only seconds to a few minutes after the exertion that prompted the attack ceases. If severe pain lasts for more than half an hour, the likelihood increases that something other than angina pectoris, perhaps a heart attack, is occurring.

Many persons, having learned the maximal activity in which they can indulge without pain, come to avoid the pain completely for long periods by restricting exercise below the critical point. Some individuals notice more difficulty with this pain during walking in the morning and can handle relatively more strenuous activity later in the day without symptoms.

**Chest Pains That Are Not Angina**

Not all chest pain is angina. Inflammation of the esophagus, the feeding tube connecting the throat to the stomach, can cause heartburn, or indigestion, symptoms that resemble angina pectoris. Such inflammation is particularly common in the individual with a hiatus hernia, a condition in which a portion of the stomach is actually above the diaphragm, in the chest. Disease of the gallbladder, peptic ulcer of the stomach or duodenum, inflammation involving the lungs, or pain in the chest wall itself can mimic angina pectoris. Typically, however, the timing, precipitating factors, character of the pain, characteristics of precipitating events, and the pattern of relief provide the physician with strong clues.

## ANGINA SUBTYPES

Angina pectoris comes in a number of forms. These include angina of effort, angina during sleep, atypical angina, intractable angina, unstable angina, and "silent" ischemic heart disease.

**Angina of Effort**

Angina of effort is the most common and distinctive form of angina and refers especially to the pain that occurs during physical activity. It may be noted especially during cold weather, during activity that has the individual raising his or her arms, during exertion after a heavy meal, or when walking up a steep incline. Occasionally, individuals will also experience the same pain during emotional crises or heated discussions, with relief when the emotional stimulus subsides or nitroglycerin is taken. One of the giants of medicine, John Hunter, who suffered from angina, complained that he was "a victim of any rogue that chooses to provoke me."

**Angina During Sleep**

In some individuals, angina occurs during the night when the individual is at rest, and without apparent cause. When a pain awakens a person from sleep, it may be difficult to exclude the possible role of a dream that had important emotional content, which the individual cannot recall. In some patients, it appears that this form is an example of atypical angina.

## Atypical Angina

Atypical, or variant, angina pectoris is angina that occurs when the individual is at rest, and without apparent provocation. This form of angina, also called Prinzmetal's angina, appears to be primarily due to spasm of the coronary arteries. Prinzmetal's angina is identified on the basis of the atypical history (pain at rest) and an electrocardiogram that shows changes different from those associated with typical angina pectoris of effort. Today treatments that are especially effective in atypical angina pectoris are available.

## Intractable Angina

The term *intractable angina* is poorly defined. In some cases, what is meant is angina that responds poorly to treatment. In other cases, it is used to denote pain that occurs frequently and with minimal provocation, so it prevents useful activity. If sleep is interrupted many times during the night, it is reasonable to call that condition intractable. The term has also been used, unfortunately, to describe unstable angina pectoris.

## Unstable Angina Pectoris

Unstable angina pectoris is a form of angina in which the pattern of angina has changed. The physical provocation required to induce the pain is often sharply reduced, and pain may occur with minimal activity or even when the person is at rest. The frequency of the attacks of pain is typically very much increased. The pain may be much less responsive to nitroglycerin and the other treatments that were effective previously. The delineation of unstable angina pectoris has been a very useful conceptual advance, since individuals with unstable angina are now recognized to be at increased risk of heart attack and now are given more definitive treatment.

## "Silent" Ischemic Heart Disease

In some circumstances, the lack of sufficient blood flow to the heart produces no pain—the ischemia is "silent." There is clear evidence that for some individuals with coronary artery disease, episodes of reduced myocardial blood flow, with electrocardiographic changes like those associated with angina, occur without accompanying pain. The precise factors responsible for the development of a low blood flow to the heart episodically and without any evidence of pain remain obscure. There are reasons for suspecting that these episodes might be important.

At the moment no cardiologist suggests that a person who does not have chest pain should have a test for "silent ischemia," unless someone who has reached middle age or older plans a dramatic increase in his or her exercise level. Thus, there is no plan to go in search of these episodes. On the other hand, for individuals who do have angina pectoris with typical episodes of chest pain, many cardiologists now have as a goal treatment that not only reduces to a minimal level or stops the eipsodes of chest pain but also minimizes episodes of silent ischemia. This is still a controversial area.

## FEATURES OF ANGINA

There are a few changes that the doctor can find on physical examination during an anginal episode; for example, blood pressure is often increased during an attack. Indeed, nitrates were first employed in the treatment of angina pectoris because a Scottish physician over a century ago noted the very hard pulse associated with an attack and thought that the administration of an agent that "softened" the pulse might be helpful. The agent that he employed, amyl nitrite, was effective in a most dramatic way. That observation led to the introduction of nitroglycerin and other nitrates for the treatment of angina.

Someone observing an individual during an attack of angina pectoris will notice a pale, strange facial expression. Often the person suffering the attack will clutch his or her chest, and a typical feature is a clenched fist. The individual will stop what he or she is doing and frequently will round his or her shoulders and perspire freely.

The electrocardiogram during an attack of angina pectoris often differs strikingly from that taken during a pain-free interval; it also differs from that taken during acute myocardial infarction.

## SPECIAL TESTS

The electrocardiogram is generally normal in the absence of an attack of chest pain, unless there has been prior injury to the heart from myocardial infarction. For this reason, a wide range of noninvasive "stress tests" have been developed, employing physical exertion to provoke an abnormality, should coronary artery disease be present. These tests were reviewed in chapter 4. Whichever test is employed, the information has several uses. A negative test, of course, reduces the likelihood that coronary artery disease is present. Should the test be positive, the amount of exercise required before provoking changes provides some insight into how much physical activity the person having a positive test can handle before provoking inadequate blood flow to the heart and symptoms.

Another important consideration is that blockage of coronary arteries at different levels might have quite different implications and lead to very different approaches to treatment. There is now universal agreement that a partial blockage of the left main coronary artery supplying much of the left ventricle is an urgent indication for surgery. A strikingly positive exercise test, especially when blood pressure falls during the test, is a clear indication that X rays of the coronary arteries will be required, and surgery is a strong likelihood.

Depending on the individual situation and the results of the exercise test, many persons with a history suggestive of coronary artery disease will undergo coronary arteriography (see chapter 4). This test reveals not only the presence, or absence, of coronary artery disease but also how many arteries are involved, where in the arteries the major disease is, and how severe the condition is. The test also provides information on the impact of the disease on ability of the heart to contract and do its job.

## LIFESTYLE CONSIDERATIONS
## WITH ANGINA

The term *medical management* indicates treatment other than a surgical procedure — treatment that may include changes in lifestyle. Smokers must give up their cigarettes. Not only is it important that they not smoke directly, but they must also avoid passive smoking—breathing smoke from someone else's cigarette.

The overweight individual imposes a substantial additional burden on the heart. Weight loss in this case is not just a reduction in the risk factor for further disease but is in fact an important part of the treatment. The physician will search for additional factors that can precipitate angina, such as anemia, an overactive thyroid gland, an infection with fever that increases heart rate, or elevated blood pressure.

For the individual with high blood pressure, treatment of the high blood pressure is an important part of the treatment of angina pectoris. Reducing the blood pressure will often reduce the frequency and severity of anginal attacks, whatever the treatment chosen. Moreover, two of the classes of agents employed for the treatment of angina pectoris are also very good at reducing blood pressure. It is good sense to select an agent that does both jobs. These agents, discussed further below, are the beta-adrenergic blocking agents and the calcium channel blocking agents.

## Change in Habits

Careful examination of the factors that precipitate an anginal attack will often provide some help in management. For the individual in whom attacks often are brought on by physical activity after a heavy meal, the obvious solution is to adjust the diet. Heavy meals can be avoided by having several smaller meals during the day. One can also change the time of one's physical activity so that heavy meals and exercise do not coincide. If exposure to cold is a provocative factor, the use of a face mask or even covering the face with a scarf can be helpful. Everyone doesn't have to move to Florida or Southern Califoria as part of his or her treatment! On the other hand, many who can afford to do so and can make the time, go to a warm climate for the worst part of the year. The impact of exposure to cold is not psychological. There is clear evidence that cold causes spasm and a reduction in blood flow to the heart.

## Physical Activity

People with angina must not consider themselves invalids. Physical activity is encouraged—the more exercise, the better.

The timing, duration, and extent of the exercise, however, must be tempered by the factors that provoke chest pain. The example of strenuous activity after a meal was cited. If walking on an upgrade or steep incline provokes chest pain, it is clearly better to walk on level ground. If climbing two flights of stairs provokes an anginal attack, it is better to climb only one. Some persons find that their ability to walk is more limited during the morning hours. If so, walk in the late afternoon, before dinner. Much of this is simple common sense, but it is surprising how often the response to exercise-provoked chest pain is to stop physical activity. Nothing could be a worse strategy for those with angina.

One of the nice by-products of physical activity is that, just as is the case for athletes, there is a conditioning process. The more physical activity an individual attempts, the more can be done in the future. On the other hand, few doctors encourage patients with angina to engage in competitive sports.

### Sexual Activity

For some time, there was a commonly held belief that patients with angina should abstain from sexual activity. This was based on the fact that in young men during sexual activity, including orgasm, blood pressure sometimes increases as much as 80 mmHg systolic and 50 mmHg diastolic, as heart rate rises to rates as high as 180 beats per minute. More recent studies have indicated that in individuals who are somewhat older, including persons with heart disease, the increase in heart rate and the increase in blood pressure are substantially less during sexual activity. This is a benefit to growing somewhat older! The equivalent physical demand is about that of climbing a flight of stairs. Moreover, the maximum period of cardiac stress lasted no more than ten or fifteen seconds in those who were middle-aged or older, again analogous to climbing a flight of stairs or performing ordinary tasks.

This information should be very reassuring, but there are some caveats. Most physicians would recommend that sexual activity not be undertaken after a heavy meal or in particular after the use of more than a little alcohol. The same applies to any physically strenuous activity.

A widely cited study from Japan of 5,559 cases of sudden death described eighteen cases of sudden death in men during sexual intercourse. There was a strikingly high frequency of extramarital sexual relations, involving much younger women and alcohol use. This information is subject to wide interpretation, since when a man dies in his matrimonial bed, there is rarely any reason for giving publicity to possible sexual context. On the other hand, the same sexual context can hardly be concealed when a married man dies while accompanied by a woman who is not his wife in surroundings far from home. It has been suggested that such a situation involves more stress, is more physically demanding, and is more likely to follow the consumption of a large amount of alcohol.

Although studies have focused on men with heart disease, the advice would surely be equally applicable to women.

## Use of Alcoholic Beverages

Again, the use of alcoholic beverages is so widespread in our society that it would seem to merit special attention. As pointed out in chapter 8, the limited use of alcohol (two three-ounce glasses of wine, one twelve-ounce bottle of beer, or one to two ounces of hard liquor) is not harmful for the individual with heart disease. Indeed, there are reasons for thinking that the impact might be salutary. The timing of alcohol consump-

**MANAGING ANGINA**

- Don't smoke.
- Avoid "passive" smoke (from others' cigarettes).
- Lose excess weight.
- Avoid heavy meals by eating three smaller meals during the day.
- Avoid combining heavy meals with exercise, including sexual activity.
- Avoid exposure to the cold (cover your face with a scarf in winter).

If you find exercise brings on chest pain, don't give up on exercise!

- Avoid strenuous activity after a meal.
- Walk later in the day instead of in the morning.
- Avoid the things that present the *most* problems (hills, too many stairs, for example).

tion is important, however. Alcohol should be avoided when one is likely to use nitroglycerin for physical activity or when one will be having a particularly large meal. There is much to be said for spreading food intake among the three meals so that the evening meal is less than most North Americans usually enjoy. In that way, the predinner cocktail or wine with dinner can be enjoyed without undue demands on the heart.

## DRUG THERAPY FOR ANGINA PECTORIS

Three classes of drugs are now widely used for the relief of angina pectoris. These drugs include nitrates, beta-adrenergic blocking agents, and calcium channel blocking agents.

### Short-acting Nitrates

A short-acting nitrate, such as nitroglycerin, has been used in the treatment of angina for over a hundred years. If the tablet is placed below the tongue and allowed to dissolve there, a beneficial response will be apparent in about two minutes on the average. The response lasts for twenty to thirty minutes. If the tablet is swallowed, there will be no benefit.

A very useful hint is to use the tablet prophylactically — that is, before one is going to perform a degree of exercise that may induce an attack of angina pectoris. For example, if walking to the bus stop involves going uphill and typically brings on an anginal attack, it is good sense to take the nigroglycerin five minutes before leaving on the walk. Too few people use this good advice.

There are few major toxic effects from nitroglycerin, though on occasion the drug may cause throbbing in the head, symptoms of giddiness, faintness, or palpitations. These symptoms usually last only a few minutes.

### Storage

When exposed to air, nitroglycerin tablets gradually lose their potency, so most physicians recommend that they be replaced every few months. A small number can be carried in a portable vial with a tight stopper and the rest left in their primary packing in the refrigerator. After a couple of days, any tablets left in the portable vial should be disposed of, as they will have lost their potency.

### Spray as an Alternative

As an alternative to the tablet placed under the tongue, a new type of delivery system based on the spraying of a measured amount of nitroglycerin into the mouth and onto the tongue has recently become available. Although the unit cost of each dose of spray is greater than the cost for tablets, the spray has some advantages, including a very rapid onset of action and a somewhat slower rate of loss of potency.

## Long-acting Nitrates

Because the relief provided by the nitroglycerin and related agents described above lasts only twenty to thirty minutes, major efforts have been made to develop nitrates that are effective for a longer period of time. The pharmaceutical industry has been successful in developing these agents by changing their primary pharmacology so that they are released much more slowly; examples are isosorbide dinitrate and pentaerythritol tetranitrate. As alternatives, special skin patches that release nitrates very gradually and nitrate paste that can be applied to the skin also have been developed.

Although widely used, these long-acting preparations share a major unfortunate characteristic. With frequent use, tolerance to their action develops rather rapidly, so a patient soon gets much less action in preventing angina pectoris.

An illustrative story provides some useful insight. People who work in the nitrate industry develop throbbing headaches when exposed to nitrates after periods of not being exposed. Tolerance reverses so rapidly that a weekend away from work is enough to make them liable to develop a headache on Monday morning. For that reason, many carry nitrates with them for the weekend and will have some nitrate in their clothes so that tolerance will not be lost. A regular daily "nitrate holiday" is a good idea. In that way, tolerance to the useful action of nitrates is less likely to develop. It is best to employ long-acting nitrates intermittently—generally during the time of peak need created by peak activity during the day.

## Beta-adrenergic Blocking Agents

Beta-adrenergic blocking agents, which block the actions of the sympathetic nerves to the heart, are very effective in reducing the frequency and severity of anginal attacks and do so through a very different mechanism than do the nitrates. The nitrates act through their action on the blood vessels. First, they dilate the coronary arteries and thus improve blood flow to the heart; second, they dilate veins so that the amount of blood in the heart is reduced. Beta-adrenergic blocking agents, on the other hand, reduce anginal frequency by reducing heart rate and by reducing the work of the heart. Since anginal pain is related to the ratio of blood supply to heart work, the fact that beta-adrenergic blockade reduces work has a favorable action.

### Advantages of Beta-adrenergic Blocking Agents
Beta-adrenergic blocking agents differ from nitrates in that they do not lose their effectiveness over time, since tolerance to them does not develop. As another dividend, their action is much longer. Some of the agents have an action that lasts twenty-four hours, so they can be employed once a day, a feature that can be very attractive.

There is another strong indication for the use of beta-blockers. A host of carefully performed trials have shown that in individuals who suffer heart attack, the likelihood of their having a recurrence of their heart attack or suffering a sudden death is decreased by about 40 percent by treatment with a beta-blocker. It does not seem to matter which beta-blocker is employed. These "secondary prevention trials" (trials designed to prevent a second attack) have made the use of a beta-adrenergic blocking agent after a heart attack almost a routine part of medical treatment (see chapter 10), unless some contraindication to such an agent is present. Many doctors believe that the evidence from the secondary prevention trials is applicable to persons with angina pectoris. They are at high risk of a heart attack, for the same reasons as are the individuals who have already had a heart attack, and the argument makes sense.

For all these reasons, beta-blockers are a mainstay in the treatment of angina pectoris. Because their mechanism of action differs from that of nitrates, the beta-blockers and nitrates are often combined in treatment. Their combined effect can be substantially greater than when they are used alone.

### Potential Problems with Beta-adrenergic Blocking Agents
What of the down side? In drug therapy, there is never an absolutely "free ride." In the case of nitrates, the problem is headache and dizziness, and tolerance. In the case of the beta-adrenergic blocking agents, there is a much longer list. In the individual who has in addition to angina pectoris a problem

When individuals have suffered a heart attack, the likelihood of their having a recurrence of their heart attack or suffering a sudden death is decreased by about 40 percent by treatment with a beta-adrenergic blocking agent.

with asthma or chronic bronchitis, the beta-blocker can provoke attacks of asthma. In the patient with borderline congestive heart failure, beta-adrenergic blockade can make the heart failure worse. In the individual with some heart block, beta-adrenergic blockade can result in complete heart block and a heart rate that is too slow to provide enough blood flow to the brain and the rest of the body. In the person who suffers from peripheral arterial disease or attacks of spasm of the fingers (Raynaud's phenomenon), the reduction of blood flow induced by beta-blockers can make the symptoms worse. These are really not side effects, in the usual sense, but rather reflect the influence of beta-adrenergic blockade that is not wanted.

As one solution, the pharmaceutical industry has developed beta-blockers that also have a feature known as intrinsic sympathomimetic activity. These beta-blockers, known as pindolol and acebutolol, have in addition to their beta-adrenergic blocking effect, an adrenalinelike action. Thus, they tend to reduce heart rate and cardiac output less and may produce less bronchial spasm. On the other hand, that influence is unpredictable, and they tend to be very expensive compared with the alternatives. For that reason, many doctors will either avoid a beta-blocker when a contraindication exists or use a very low dose.

### Generic Beta-adrenergic Blocking Agents

One of the first of the beta-adrenergic blocking agents, propranolol, has recently become a generic. Several pharmaceutical firms now market generic propranolol; the cost runs about half of the original propranolol and about half of the other beta-blockers. What is the down side of these agents?

The beta-blockers that followed propranolol were developed to have several features that differ from propranolol. Propranolol is nonselective; it blocks the receptors in the heart to the same degree that it blocks receptors in the lung, that are responsible for asthma. Some agents (metoprolol tartrate and atenolol) have been developed that are beta-1 selective—they

---

**PROBLEMS THAT CAN BE AGGRAVATED BY BETA-ADRENERGIC BLOCKING AGENTS**

-Asthma
-Chronic bronchitis
-Borderline congestive heart failure
-Heart block
-Peripheral arterial disease or Raynaud's phenomenon

---

block the receptors in the heart more effectively than they block the receptors in the lung. Although much has been made of it in a marketing sense, the difference is too small to matter and to be worth the difference in price for most people.

Another feature of some of the newer drugs is the intrinsic sympathomimetic activity described earlier (see page 149). That can be useful to the occasional individual, but again the price differential is generally too much to pay. It is only for the occasional person who benefits sufficiently that these more expensive agents should be considered.

### Propranolol and Mood

Perhaps the most important difference between propranolol and some of the new drugs is that propranolol is much more soluble in fat than most of the other beta-blockers. At the other extreme, there are some that are much more soluble in water, such as nadolol and atenolol. This is important, since the brain has fat as its major constituent; propranolol, because of its greater lipid solubility, will reach the brain in much higher concentrations.

Depression, extreme disturbances in sleep patterns leading to vivid and unpleasant dreams and nightmares, and impotence are more frequent with propranolol than with the other beta-blockers. On the other hand, for the individual who has anxiety as a frequent problem and in whom anxiety provokes anginal attacks, this action of propranolol on the brain can be very useful, as it results in reduced anxiety.

For the person who is depressed or who has problems with sleep patterns or for a man who is having sexual difficulties, propranolol can tip the balance in the wrong way. For the person who has none of these problems, the generic agent is a very good choice. The reduction in cost is associated only with a small reduction in convenience—generic propanolol must be taken three or four times a day. For many individuals, though, the price of an alternative is worth paying.

## Calcium Channel Blocking Agents

The third major class of drug employed for the treatment of angina pectoris is the calcium channel blocking agent (calcium blocker). The movement of calcium from the bloodstream to the inside of smooth muscle cells in the blood vessel wall is required for contraction. The calcium channel blocking agents prevent coronary artery spasm by preventing that movement of calcium, and thus the spasm. A vast body of information makes it clear that they improve blood flow to the heart.

These drugs were introduced well after the beta-blockers and have almost caught up with them in the frequency of their use in the United States. They have been used for much longer in Europe. If nitrates were the wonder drugs of a hundred years ago and beta-blockers the wonder drugs of the late sixties and early seventies, the calcium blockers can be considered the wonder drugs of the early eighties for angina pectoris.

The calcium blockers differ from the beta-blockers in ways other than their mechanism of action. There are small differences in the structure and characteristics of the beta-adrenergic blocking agents. The three currently available calcium channel blocking agents in the United States—verapamil, nifedipine, and diltiazem—differ in their chemical structure, the site at which they act, and in some of their side effects.

### Side Effects of Verapamil, Nifedipine, and Diltiazem

Verapamil tends to produce constipation, which can be a substantial problem—especially for those who already have trouble with their bowel habit. Estimates indicate that 5 to 20 percent of individuals taking verapamil could have such a problem.

Nifedipine tends to produce many of the vasodilator side effects that were seen with the nitrates, including vascular throbbing headache, flushing, and fast heart rate. Although some tolerance may develop to these side effects, they are the most common reason that persons discontinue nifedipine use. Another problem with nifedipine is the tendency for some persons to develop swollen ankles, sufficiently severe that fitting shoes may be a problem. For obvious reasons, related to their cosmetic effect, men appear to handle this side effect better than women. As opposed to the ankle swelling that occurs in heart failure and that reflects retention of sodium and water, this swelling does not reflect that retention but rather an action on the blood vessels. Elevation can be helpful in reversing the swelling, but many people give up on the drug nevertheless. A new formulation of nifedipine that reduces the frequency and severity of some of these side effects and some new drugs that are similar to nifedipine and appear to have a longer action and perhaps fewer side effects may soon be available. They are not currently marketed.

Diltiazem, the third calcium channel blocking agent, is the most recently introduced and appears to induce fewer of the vasodilator side effects than does nifedipine. It does not cause constipation.

### Greatest Impact of Calcium Channel Blocking Agents

Some patients with angina pectoris do not respond to beta-blockers with improvement. Indeed, both the frequency and severity of the attacks of angina may be increased with a beta-blocker. There is strong reason for believing that such persons have spasm of the coronary artery as the major factor causing the anginal attack, and beta-blockers may make spasm more severe. This sequence of events is more likely to occur in those with atypical or variant angina pectoris. It is especially for such persons that the calcium blockers have had their largest impact. When anginal pain is induced by coronary artery spasm, treatment with a calcium channel blocking agent can be almost magical and is especially dramatic when nitrates and beta-blockers have been essentially ineffective.

### Potential Problems of Calcium Channel Blocking Agents

There are many fewer contraindications to calcium blockers than to beta-blockers. For the individual with some heart block, a cardiac arrhythmia that leads to a very slow heart

---

**CALCIUM CHANNEL BLOCKING AGENTS—POSSIBLE SIDE EFFECTS**

Verapamil: constipation
Nifedipine: headache, flushing, fast heart rate, swollen ankles
Diltiazem: headache, flushing, swollen ankles

rate, nifedipine is a better choice of calcium channel blocking drug, since it tends to increase heart rate whereas the other two drugs decrease it. For the patient with borderline congestive heart failure, nifedipine is again probably better tolerated.

Because of the increase in heart rate induced by nifedipine, many physicians prefer to combine a beta-blocking drug with nifedipine than with the other two calcium channel blocking drugs, since beta-blockers tend to reduce heart rate. On the other hand, experienced physicians will often combine one of the other calcium channel blocking drugs with the beta-blockers.

The disadvantage of calcium blockers is cost. As a group, these drugs are substantially more expensive than are the beta-blockers and the nitrates. Price competition and patent expiration have led to a somewhat lower price for verapamil than for the other two.

### Combinations of Drugs

Today, physicians have come to recognize that obstruction that is purely mechanical, on the one hand, and spasm with little mechanical obstruction, on the other, are both possible (see page 112). Many individuals, in fact, have some combination of obstruction and spasm. Hence, both a beta-blocker and a calcium blocker are commonly used in the patient with typical angina pectoris.

## COMBINATIONS OF THERAPY

General health measures involving cigarettes, fitness, and weight loss and the three classes of drugs should not be seen as alternatives. General health measures should be undertaken by everyone.

Most physicians today recommend that combinations of the drugs be employed. Perhaps the most common combination would be intermittent nitrate use, along with beta-adrenergic blockade—or, for the person for whom a beta-adrenergic blocking agent is either ineffective or contraindicated, a calcium channel blocking agent. A substantial number of persons now receive all three classes of drugs. Indeed, there are individuals with difficult angina in whom the combination of nifedipine and diltiazem—two calcium blockers—is effective when neither was effective when used alone.

Medical therapy—here, mainly new drugs and new ways to use drugs—is much more effective today than it was as recently as five years ago. There is a clearer understanding of the condition and the changes in lifestyle needed to improve or alleviate it.

## Medicine in the Morning

Precisely when a person takes his or her medicine is too infrequently addressed, and there is growing evidence that it merits attention. A number of studies have now suggested that there is a peak frequency of sudden death, heart attack, and stroke that occurs in the morning, and particularly shortly after rising from bed. The reason for that frequency is obscure, but several possibilities are being considered, including the rise in blood pressure that occurs when a person gets out of bed, increased sympathetic nervous system activity related to the physical activity, and some recent evidence that the platelets are more sticky at that time—perhaps related to sympathetic nervous system activity. Whatever the explanation, most treatment regimens have not been designed to cover the morning interval; the effects of drugs tend to wear off during the night, and the precise timing of the morning medication often tends to be haphazard.

There are no studies to indicate that the precise time of taking one's medication in the morning will change these peak frequencies of heart attack, stroke, and sudden death. Such studies are complicated and difficult to design and perform, so the answers will not be in for many years. On the other hand, since it is so very easy to leave a glass of water and your medication next to the bed, and since there is no risk to taking the medication when you first awake, why not do so? If taking the medication as soon as you wake up becomes a routine part of your life, you are also more likely to remember to take your medication.

## Aspirin Use

Aspirin is not a treatment for angina pectoris but rather a treatment for complications of atherosclerosis. The first step in the formation of a blood clot when the blood vessel wall is abnormal involves the deposit of sticky platelets on the surface of the blood vessel. Aspirin acts to reduce platelet stickiness, thus reducing the likelihood that a clot will form. In the case of unstable angina pectoris, the use of aspirin is especially important because there is evidence that a large percentage of people with unstable angina are at immediate risk of heart attack, and clot formation plays a role.

What dose of aspirin is best? This is a situation in which less is better. Although some studies have shown that four regular aspirin a day will be effective, there is evidence to suggest that lower doses are better. Thus, one aspirin a day or even one baby aspirin a day is probably the best choice. In some studies, one 350 mg aspirin taken every other day has been effective, and this might be the preferred way to use aspirin.

## INTERVENTIONAL TREATMENTS

Beyond medical therapy, two interventional maneuvers are useful in treating angina pectoris. These are coronary artery bypass surgery and percutaneous transluminal coronary angioplasty.

### Surgical Treatment

In the past four decades, there have been numerous surgical methods devised to provide a new blood supply to the heart. For the past decade, the most direct surgical approach to providing an arterial blood supply to the heart has been either endarterectomy, which means repairing the damaged coronary artery by removing the injured lining, or bypass grafting. In the case of the bypass graft, a connection is made between the aorta or another large artery and the coronary blood vessels downstream from the area of obstruction. The bypass may be made by moving an artery from the chest wall, the internal mammary artery, to the coronary artery beyond the obstruction (see figure 18), or by the use of a piece of vein from the individual's leg (the saphenous vein) to connect the aorta to the coronary artery beyond the obstruction (see figure 19) or the use of some artificial material such as Dacron® to accomplish the same goal.

#### Choosing Surgery

Until recently, the most clear indication that surgery was required was failure of medical therapy. The individual whose life had become intolerable because of continued pain provoked by even minimal activity often would choose to have a surgi-

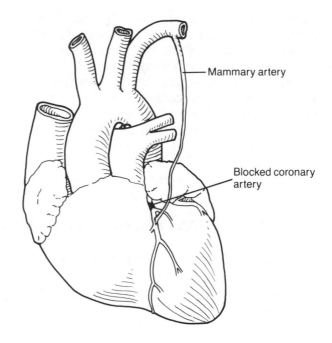

Mammary artery

Blocked coronary
artery

**Figure 18.   Mammary Arterial Bypass Graft**

The mammary artery, normally found along the rib cage, is used to bypass a coronary blockage. It remains attached to its own blood supply at the top end. This type of graft may last longer and do somewhat better than when a leg vein is used for the bypass.

cal procedure, despite the risk. Surgery as an alternative became progressively more attractive as the risk of surgery came down. With experience in the anesthetic procedure and the increase in technical facility with the surgery itself, the risk is down to a surprisingly low 1 to 3 percent in experienced hands—surprisingly low in view of the severity of the primary illness.

As a goal of surgery, the relief of symptoms obviously had great merit, but there was always a second consideration. Could one change the natural progression of coronary artery disease, delaying death, by performing the surgical procedure? The first group of individuals in whom a change in progression was identified were those at greatest risk, for the obvious reason: the greater the risk, the easier it is to prove that one has reduced the risk.

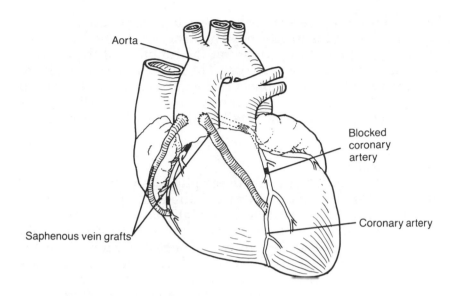

**Figure 19.   Saphenous Vein Grafts**

The saphenous vein is taken from a leg and used to bypass a blocked coronary artery by attaching one end to the aorta and the other end to the coronary artery beyond the obstruction. This has been the most widely used operation to bypass obstructed coronary arteries.

The person who has an obstruction of the large coronary artery at the origin of the coronary arterial tree—known as left main disease to physicians—has a very large part of the heart at risk should a clot form. People with obstruction are so likely to suffer sudden death, or a very rapid and difficult downhill course, when their partially obstructed artery becomes occluded that they require surgical treatment urgently. Such individuals are often identified during stress testing and today never have a trial of medical therapy.

The publication of several studies in which medical therapy and surgery were compared has provided some insight into who is likely to benefit from surgery rather than medical therapy, not so much in terms of symptoms but rather in terms of long-term outcome. Perhaps the most important source of information has been the CASS (Coronary Artery Surgery Study) study recently completed in the United States and widely publicized in the press. Although there are numerous caveats, in general, the individual most likely to benefit from surgery is the one with more severe disease—two or three coronary arteries involved with an advanced obstruction, rather than one, therefore enough obstruction that the function of the heart is moderately reduced even at rest. The information, then, from the more recent studies supports strongly what might have been anticipated. The more severe the disease, the more likely it is that surgery is better than medical therapy alone at prolonging life.

### Age and Surgery

One of the questions that many physicians and, of course, their patients have been concerned about involves the age of the person coming to surgery. One might have anticipated that the older the individual, the less likely it was that surgery would be better than medical therapy when longevity after treatment was the goal. In fact, for those at high risk, even individuals over the age of seventy-five have shown substantial benefit from surgery. Increasing age is not an absolute contraindication to surgery.

There is an additional caveat. Unless the risk factors for atherosclerosis are dealt with effectively, the disease in the native arteries and in the bypassed artery tends to progress. With many years of experience with bypass surgery, physicians are now seeing many individuals who have had bypass surgery some years ago, with success. Over the years, however, the original disease has progressed—as has the disease in the bypassed vessel itself—and, as a result, the person once more is a candidate for surgery. Surgery, the second time around, is technically much more difficult. For this reason, many doctors are suggesting that the initial surgery be delayed whenever possible.

## Percutaneous Transluminal Coronary Angioplasty

This technique was described in chapter 4 (see pages 52–53). Rather than performing a surgical procedure to bypass or repair the damaged artery, a special catheter is used to open the artery. The catheter that is used has a balloon at its end that can be inflated in the narrowed segment to dilate it and restore blood flow (see figure 20). The rapid development of this technique has been one of the most exciting chapters in the story of coronary artery disease. When Dr. Andreas Gruntzig of Switzerland first described the method in the late 1970s, only about 15 percent of patients with coronary artery disease had a lesion (an abnormal change in a coronary artery) that could

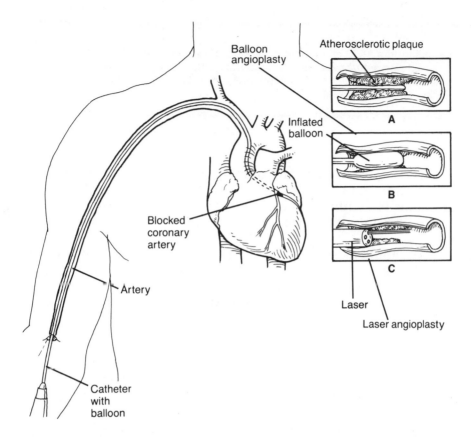

**Figure 20. Angioplasty Applied to the Coronary Artery**

A catheter introduced into an artery in the forearm has been placed in the coronary artery **(A)** with a balloon strategically located so that when it is inflated, it opens a partially closed coronary artery **(B)**. A research procedure involving replacement of a balloon with a laser **(C)** is shown. The laser can cause the disappearance of the occluding atherosclerotic plaque. Although lasers are not in common use today, and are still the subject of research, many experts believe that they are the technique of the future.

be treated in this way because of technical limitations. Over the past few years, the equipment available and the technical facility in using it have advanced so rapidly that the percentage of individuals who can benefit from angioplasty has increased tremendously. At one time, angioplasty of only one lesion in an individual could be attempted, and then only if the lesion was in a special location. Today, many more lesions in many more patients can be treated successfully.

According to a 1983 study by the National Heart, Lung and Blood Institute, about 60 percent of patients with moderate angina report that during the first year after surgery their pain is completely relieved. Fifty percent remain free of the pain five years later.

The advantages of angioplasty are obvious. Because it is unnecessary to open the chest, the number of complications are sharply reduced. The cost is substantially lower as well. Many individuals are up and around within a few days.

As should now be evident, there are many effective options for the treatment of angina pectoris. Treatment has two goals: relief of chest pain and prevention of a heart attack, or myocardial infarction, described in the next chapter.

# 10

## The Heart Attack—
## Acute Myocardial Infarction

As heart disease is now the acknowledged greatest single cause of death in this country, so the heart attack is the most common cause of heart damage. Sudden obstruction of a coronary artery (acute coronary occlusion) is caused, typically, by the development of a blood clot on an injured part of the lining of the artery (coronary thrombosis). The term *myocardial infarction* implies the death (necrosis) of a portion of the heart muscle because of a complete or nearly complete interruption of its blood supply.

### SYMPTOMS

In most individuals, acute myocardial infarction produces a distinctive series of abnormalities. The characteristics include pain in the chest that is similar in location and radiation to that of angina pectoris but differs in its greater severity and duration, its usual independence from exercise, and its resistance to nitroglycerin. Generally a person having a heart attack feels more sick than does the individual with angina pectoris, and fever and other signs of a systemic reaction to the damaged tissue are frequent.

By no means everyone who has a myocardial infarction experiences this process. In some large epidemiological studies, in which serial electrocardiograms were performed over several years, it was found that up to 25 percent of cases of acute myocardial infarction had occurred without any symptoms. This less typical process was more common in patients with diabetes, presumably because of the impact of diabetes on the nerves to the heart, but was not restricted to them. Estimates indicate that about a third of the individuals who die suddenly, without any symptoms, do so because of acute coronary thrombosis and disruption of heart function.

The contributory and predisposing factors to acute coronary thrombosis are essentially identical to those described for atherosclerosis (chapters 7 and 8), and angina pectoris (chapter 9). What differs in acute myocardial infarction is that complete or near complete obstruction of the artery results in the destruction of heart tissue (see figure 21).

## WHAT PRECIPITATES
## THE HEART ATTACK

Studies of patients' activities immediately preceding a heart attack have noted physical exercise and even moderate or usual exertion in only a small fraction prior to the beginning of pain. In this way, myocardial infarction differs from typical angina pectoris. On the other hand, the peak frequency shortly after

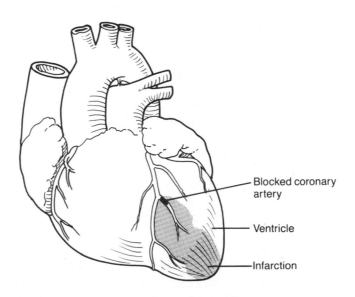

**Figure 21.  Myocardial Infarction Caused by Blockage of a
             Major Coronary Artery**

Because the blood supply to the top of the ventricle was inadequate, the area underwent infarction.

arising suggests that hormonal and other factors related to the change from the sleep to physically active stage of the day might play a more important role in heart attack.

However, there are enough cases of acute myocardial infarction that occur during unusually demanding physical activity—someone who is out of condition shoveling snow from a driveway after a storm is a common example—that the individual at risk of a heart attack must use good judgment in handling these situations. They are best avoided unless one knows that one is sufficiently fit to handle them.

There are rare causes of acute myocardial infarction, such as inflammation of the arteries, which can occur elsewhere in the circulatory system, or congenital abnormalities of the arteries, but they are very uncommon.

## DIAGNOSIS—AT THE HOSPITAL

Suspicion of acute myocardial infarction mandates a trip to a hospital emergency room—by ambulance, if necessary, so that oxygen can be administered en route if needed. There the tests required to establish the diagnosis can be performed quickly, and treatment can be instituted. The electrocardiogram remains a most important element in the diagnosis. Characteristic abnormalities of the electrocardiogram are important both for the detection of a myocardial infarction and to determine its location and extent. If the area in jeopardy is large and extends throughout the full thickness of the heart, diagnosis is generally straightforward. If the area in jeopardy is smaller, the changes may be much more nonspecific. When myocardial tissue is damaged, certain chemicals, called enzymes, within the cells are released into the bloodstream, and their measurement in serum provides clear evidence that infarction has occurred, and even an index as to how much tissue is damaged or destroyed.

In general, changes both in the electrocardiogram and especially in the enzymes may not be evident for six to eight hours. This explains the frequent necessity for a person with chest pain to remain in limbo in an emergency room until a clear yes or no can be determined from the tests. Indeed the problem is so common that many hospitals have developed "holding units" as a satellite to the emergency room so that individuals with a potentially transient problem can avoid the administration aspects of hospitalization and yet be under surveillance.

**EXAMPLES OF ECG READINGS**

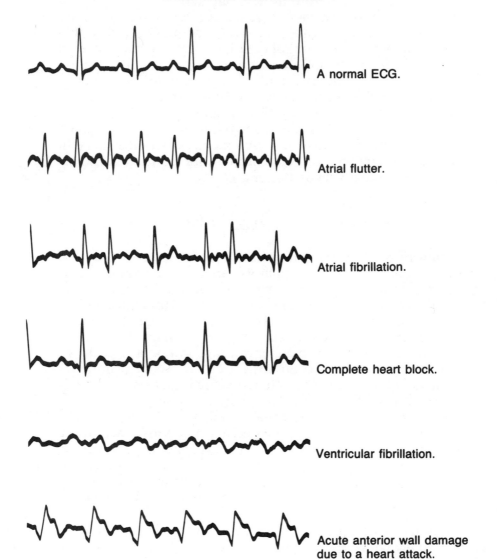

A normal ECG.

Atrial flutter.

Atrial fibrillation.

Complete heart block.

Ventricular fibrillation.

Acute anterior wall damage
due to a heart attack.

Acute posterior wall damage
due to a heart attack.

## IMMEDIATE TREATMENT

If the tests are positive, hospital admission is routine. There treatment for the pain can be undertaken along with continuous monitoring for cardiac arrhythmias. The rhythm of the heart's pumping action is coordinated by electrical signals carried in the heart's cells. Damage to cells can disrupt the heart's rhythm. Some abnormality of cardiac rhythm occurs in a substantial fraction of patients experiencing acute myocardial infarction, and many abnormalities require treatment with one or more antiarrhythmic agents during the first several days (see chapter 12).

The fundamental philosophy of the treatment of acute myocardial infarction has evolved over the past two decades. As recently as twenty years ago, admission to a hospital for a heart attack meant that the patient would remain for four to six weeks, much of that time in bed. The rationale for that approach involved the belief that the injured area had to heal completely, to a strong scar, before physical activity could be allowed.

Physicians now recognize, on the basis of unequivocal information from a wide variety of studies, that that approach was not only unnecessary but indeed contributed substantially to a widespread lack of well-being of individuals after heart attacks. Prolonged bed rest can convert any healthy person into an invalid who is weak, tires easily, has a poor bowel habit, and feels dizzy while walking.

Today the person with an uncomplicated myocardial infarction is rarely in the hospital for more than two weeks, and physical activity is allowed earlier.

There are so many effective treatments for cardiac arrhythmias today that they rarely represent a critical factor in survival. What is probably the critical element in long-term survival is the amount of tissue destroyed. In individuals with a very tiny myocardial infarction, once cardiac arrhythmias have been dealt with, the likelihood is the person will have an uncomplicated course in the hospital and go back to a normal or near normal life. A very large infarct can result in severe congestive heart failure, shock, or death. For that reason, substantial efforts are made to limit the size of myocardial infarction.

There is one important exception to the rule that smaller infarcts do better than larger ones once arrhythmias have been dealt with. In the case of myocardial infarction in which damage threatens only the inner portion of the heart wall, the result is likely to be a smaller infarct. Despite this, evidence has

Prolonged bed rest can convert any healthy person into an invalid. Today the individual with an uncomplicated heart attack is rarely in the hospital for more than two weeks.

accumulated that this class of infarct in particular is likely to extend in the first several days after the acute event. For that reason, special approaches have been devised for the treatment of this class of infarct.

## Agents That Diminish Damage

General care for acute myocardial infarction includes bed rest, the provision of oxygen where necessary, the treatment of chest pain, and the treatment of cardiac arrhythmias.

For the patient with an acute myocardial infarction that does not extend through the full thickness of the heart wall, there is recent evidence that one can reduce the likelihood of extension of the infarction by treatment with a calcium channel blocking agent, diltiazem (see chapter 9).

Major emphasis is now being given to attempts to reverse thrombosis through the administration of an agent that can dissolve the blood clot in the coronary artery. Some agents such as streptokinase and urokinase have been available for this purpose for some time. When streptokinase is infused directly into the coronary artery so that very high concentrations can be achieved there, it has been possible to dissolve the clot and restore blood flow to the heart in a remarkable percentage of individuals—over 80 percent. When this is accomplished in the first four hours or so after the onset of chest pain, the result has often been the restoration of a normal or near normal area of heart muscle. The myocardial infarction has been averted.

Of course, to achieve that goal, it was necessary to get the individuals suffering the coronary thrombosis to a well-equipped and well-staffed special laboratory during the critical interval. To place a catheter in the coronary artery required the special expertise and facilities needed for coronary arteriography. Although widely successful in a limited number of centers, this approach was not generalized, and cannot be. To give these agents intravenously and have them as successful in reversing the clot in the coronary artery, much higher doses would be required, so the risk of hemorrhage would go up substantially. For that reason, when given intravenously, lower streptokinase doses were employed and the success rate was lower.

### The Promise of TPA

The obvious answer was to find an agent that would be effective in thrombolysis (dissolving clots) and that would be more specific for a freshly formed clot in an artery, such as the coronary artery, with little action elsewhere. This would reduce the danger of hemorrhage. Some great medical detective work and brilliant science has indeed identified such an agent. The agent is called tissue plasminogen activator (TPA). TPA does not dissolve a clot directly but rather activates a normal enzyme in the blood at the surface of a clot so that the thrombolysis occurs in the area of the clot and nowhere else. Of course, if one has a clot that is preventing hemorrhage elsewhere, for example in the brain, that clot will also be dissolved, and cerebral hemorrhage can occur. Despite that limitation, the specificity of TPA is obviously greater than that of the earlier clot-dissolving agents.

Studies to see whether the intravenous administration of TPA will change the natural course of coronary thrombosis are ongoing. The early results are certainly promising, and there is substantial excitement about the promise of this approach. Intravenous administration, of course, does not require the special facilities needed to administer a drug directly into the coronary artery, so treatment can be undertaken anywhere, day or night.

Once the clot has been dissolved, the reason for the clot formation that led to the risk of acute myocardial infarction remains. The available approaches to reduce risk include coronary angioplasty and surgery. Effective clot dissolution has sharply reduced the amount of heart irreversibly damaged because of insufficient blood supply.

---

Studies are currently ongoing to see whether TPA will change the natural course of coronary thrombosis. There is substantial excitement about the promise of this approach.

## FACTORS CRITICAL TO SURVIVAL

There is an enormous range of outcomes from acute myocardial infarction. As pointed out earlier, a small percentage of individuals will die immediately upon coronary thrombosis, many never experiencing pain. Others develop serious cardiac arrhythmias en route to the hospital, so for many centers, monitoring for cardiac arrhythmias is routinely performed in the ambulance. The emergency team in the ambulance has the experience and the medications to treat such arrhythmias.

## RECOVERY AFTER THE HEART ATTACK

It is now fairly common, and in many centers routine, to attempt to assess the status of the individual in two to four weeks after acute myocardial infarction. The approaches include ambulatory electrocardiograph monitoring with a Holter monitor (chapter 4) and exercise testing (chapter 4). In this way, individuals who are at very low risk of further trouble can be so informed and their rehabilitation program enhanced. People who have increased risk are identified so measures can be undertaken to prevent recurrent problems.

Rehabilitation begins in the hospital. Physicians now avoid prolonged immobilization as much as possible. Formal exercise (stress) testing often helps determine what exercise regimen is best and what can be handled. In the first few weeks, low work loads are allowed, including activities required to take care of one's self, walking, and perhaps some easy exercising involving mild calisthenics. Thereafter, a graded exercise program is often undertaken. Increasing levels of activity result in a progressively greater level of physical fitness. After three months, many persons can participate in high-level calisthenics and moderately high level endurance exercises.

Secondary prevention of myocardial infarction with beta-adrenergic blocking agents in survivors of myocardial infarction was mentioned in chapter 9. They are now widely employed for this purpose. Beta-adrenergic blockade can make exercise somewhat more difficult, but there is clear evidence that beta-adrenergic blockade does not limit the ability of an exercise program to improve fitness.

There is substantial overlap in the approach to the patient following acute myocardial infarction and the treatment of angina pectoris. For reasons described in chapter 9, a substantial number of individuals may have coronary artery bypass surgery or coronary angioplasty.

## LIFE AFTER RECOVERY

To prevent further trouble, careful attention to the risk factors described in chapter 8 is an absolute requirement. Many doctors have noted that the warning provided by a heart attack often provides the stimulus for survivors to change their lifestyles.

The goal of medicine today is to accomplish more than relief of symptoms and prevention of death and disability. For those who have had heart attacks, the quality of life after recovery and the resumption of normal activity are also important goals. The entire logic of the new approach to the heart attack has been to provide a life as near normal as possible. Doctors rarely advise those who have had heart attacks to give up their employment. Their return to work is an important part of recovery. Fortunately, there are only a few occupations—such as airline pilot, fire fighter, or police officer—in which an acute myocardial infarction precludes continuation of employment. Employers in these fields are sensitive to this issue and often can find alternative but gratifying work for individuals who have had a heart attack.

Most physicians agree that most people who survive an acute myocardial infarction are not invalids. This is a message as important to family members as it is to the individual who has had the infarct.

# 11

# Heart Failure

Perhaps the most widely misunderstood term among nonmedical persons is *heart failure*. One can have heart disease and not have heart failure. One can have a heart attack and not have heart failure. Indeed, under some unusual circumstances, one can have heart failure despite the fact that the heart has no intrinsic structural abnormality. What is this puzzling thing called heart failure?

The primary function of the heart is to serve as a pump. When the heart is unable to meet the demands made of it, to provide an adequate blood flow to all the organs in the body, the result is congestive heart failure.

Let us begin with a physical analogy—a mechanical pump. One can use any mechanical pump in two ways. First, one can use a pump with the primary purpose of moving fluid *from* a place. Anyone who has had pipes burst or a sewer plugged and has used a pump to keep the accumulation of fluid out of the basement knows that purpose well. On the other hand, one can use a pump to move fluid *to* a place. Anyone who has used a pump to spray insecticide on trees knows that purpose equally well. In the first case, the pump fails if it cannot keep up with the accumulation of water in the basement. In the second case, the pump fails to do the job if the area to be sprayed extends beyond the region of the pump.

In the case of heart failure, both of these problems arise. First, the heart is incompetent to keep up with the return of blood in the circulatory system, so the blood is dammed up. Second, the heart is inadequate to provide all the blood flow required by the various organs in the body, especially when demand for blood flow increases as it does during exercise.

**171**

## CAUSES OF HEART FAILURE

Any kind of injury to the heart can make it inadequate as a pump and can thus lead to heart failure. One obvious and very common example is the heart attack, described in chapter 10. If sufficient damage to enough heart muscle occurs, the heart's efficiency as a pump is lessened substantially. If the pressure against which the heart has to work is increased extremely, as occurs in severe hypertension (see chapter 5), once again the result may be heart failure. Inflammation of the heart muscle (myocarditis) or injury to the heart muscle (cardiomyopathy) can also cause heart failure.

Rheumatic heart disease was once a very important cause of congestive heart failure, through progressive destruction of the heart valves. As a consequence, the valves might become very rigid, obstructing blood flow through them. Another consequence of rheumatic fever was a leaky valve. In either case, the efficiency of the heart as a pump could be reduced sharply even though the heart muscle was intact. Rheumatic heart disease is a consequence of streptococcal infection. Fortunately, rheumatic heart has become a progressively more uncommon cause of heart failure, at least in part because of the development of antibiotics that allow physicians to treat streptococcal infection effectively.

Congenital heart disease, abnormality in the heart and main vessels that an individual is born with, was also a common cause of heart failure in the past (see figure 22). This is now less common with better prenatal care. In addition, there are now excellent surgical procedures to deal with many of the common congenital problems.

The demand made on the heart is an important variable. If a person has severe anemia, severe hypertension, or a hole between an artery and a vein (arteriovenous aneurysm) so that large volumes of blood are being pumped from the artery to the veins without reaching any tissue, the heart may be no match for the demands made on it. A severely overactive thyroid or a specific vitamin deficiency (beriberi) can lead to heart failure despite a relatively intact heart. In the case of the severely overactive thyroid gland, each tissue is operating at a higher metabolic rate, and very inefficiently, so the demands for blood flow are increased sharply.

Thiamine is a vitamin critical for efficient metabolism. In the case of thiamine deficiency, which leads to beriberi heart disease, the result is similar to that associated with too much thyroid activity. An inefficient metabolic system demands more blood flow. Heavy physical demands, such as lifting and carrying, also put a major burden on the heart.

A particularly striking example follows: A young Eskimo who lived in the far North and worked as a trapper was hurrying home for Christmas, walking on snowshoes (which is physically very demanding) and carrying a 140-pound pack of furs on his back. Because he was late for Christmas dinner, he chose to hurry up a moderately steep incline for several miles in the cold. The result was his first, and a very sudden, attack of heart failure. After emergency treatment, and with some rest, there was absolutely no residual sign of heart failure. He did have an abnormality of his aortic valve that was related to earlier rheumatic heart disease. Only under very special circumstances did this abnormality make the pump function inadequate. Under ordinary, everyday circumstances, his heart was fully competent.

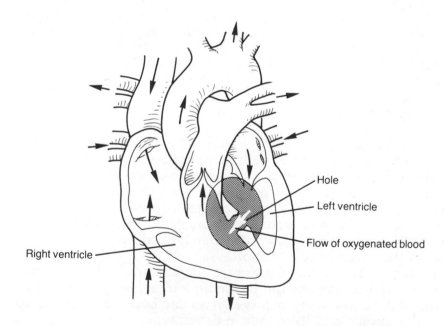

**Figure 22.   Congential Heart Disease Due to Ventricular Septal Defect**
With this abnormality, there is a hole between the right and left ventricles, so oxygenated blood flows from the left to the right. Although congenital heart disease is usually diagnosed in younger persons, on occasion adults are found to have heart problems related to congenital heart disease.

## SYMPTOMS OF HEART FAILURE

The two actions of the pump, those that are primarily "backward" (that involve removing fluid from somewhere), and those that are primarily "forward" (that involve delivering fluid somewhere), both contribute to the symptoms and findings in heart failure.

### Difficulty in Breathing

The backward failure results in accumulation of blood and fluid in the veins and tissues. Accumulation of fluid in the lungs results in difficulty in breathing, which is typically worse when the individual lies down. The reason that breathing is more difficult when lying down is that blood is trapped in the veins of the bowel and in the legs by gravity when a person is sitting or standing and shifts into the chest when the person lies down. When people find that they feel uncomfortable unless they are propped up by several pillows when they go to sleep (orthopnea), it is an early symptom of heart failure. Occasionally, individuals find that they wake up from a deep sleep very short of breath (paroxysmal nocturnal dyspnea). In their panic, they leap from bed—which moves the blood from their chest to their abdomen and legs and quickly reverses the shortness of breath.

### Swelling Due to Fluid Retention

Ankle swelling (edema), which can progress to swelling of the entire body (anasarca), reflects retention of sodium and chloride by the kidneys. For many people, ankle swelling is the first symptom of heart failure, especially when the heart failure has occurred very gradually rather than abruptly. When heart failure occurs abruptly (acute pulmonary edema), shortness of breath—again generally worse when lying down—is almost always the major manifestation.

When the backward pressure and accumulation of fluid is severe, there may be fluid in the abdomen (ascites) and function of the chronically engorged liver can become impaired, so mild jaundice and liver failure develop.

### Reduced Activity

The forward manifestations of heart failure reflect an inadequate ability of the heart to maintain blood flow. This is most evident when an individual tries to be active. People with heart failure will often avoid stairs and will reduce their physical activity in most ways. Indeed, the reduction in physical activity can occur so gradually they may be unaware of the fact that they have narrowed their lives around their reduced physical capacity. Formal exercise (stress) tests, for example, often show that people with heart failure become exhausted by walking much more easily than they did before, in spite of the fact that they did not notice the decrease in stamina themselves. Another manifestation of inadequate blood flow, especially when heart failure is severe, is an abnormality in kidney function. Reduced blood flow to the kidneys probably causes them to retain sodium, which contributes to edema, shortness of breath, and other manifestations of heart failure.

## GENERAL MANAGEMENT OF HEART FAILURE

When heart failure is severe, or comes on quickly and unexpectedly without a prior history of heart disease, the place for treatment is a hospital. There, initial treatment can be undertaken, both to relieve symptoms and to improve the function of the heart. The tests required to determine whether more definitive treatment is possible can then be undertaken.

### Bed Rest

Bed rest, to relieve symptoms, is a critical factor in the early treatment of heart failure. Bed rest during the *early* management of heart failure reduces the work of the heart. With time, restriction of physical activity is modified so as to disturb the individual's lifestyle as little as possible.

### Improving the Pump

A second approach to managing heart failure involves improving the ability of the heart to function as a pump. The drug digitalis has been recognized in this role for over two hundred years and remains an important element in treatment today. Treatment with digitalis can be initiated for those who have never received it before. For persons who have already been on digitalis, measurement of plasma concentrations of digitalis often makes it possible to adjust the dose. Both too much and too little digitalis can be a problem; the drug has a narrow margin of safety. There are a number of research drugs currently under investigation that are also designed to improve the pumping quality of the heart, and one has been approved for short-term emergency use in heart failure.

If the pump's inadequate function reflects too slow or too rapid a heart rate, drugs are available to correct the rate and rhythm of the heart, thereby improving heart function. If heart block, a cardiac arrhythmia that results in a very slow heart rate, is a problem, the physician may wish to insert an electrical pacemaker to regulate the rate of heart contraction. This is a device that can substitute for the natural group of cells that automatically generate the needed impulses for contraction. External pacemakers are also available. (See chapter 12.)

### Reducing the Heart's Work Load

The work load of the heart is reduced initially by bed rest. Attention to other details such as correction of anemia or of overactive thyroid function will also reduce the burden on the pump. So will losing weight, if obesity is a problem.

Part of the work of the heart is overcoming the pressure in the large arteries so that the heart can empty itself of blood. It has long been recognized that reducing blood pressure in someone with hypertension improves the function of his or her heart. It has more recently been recognized that drugs that dilate small arteries also reduce the work of the heart in someone whose blood pressure is normal. At the moment, only one class of drugs, the converting enzyme inhibitors, is approved by the FDA for treatment of heart failure, though others also have been found useful under some circumstances. Exciting recent news is that the converting enzyme inhibitors, captopril and enalapril (discussed in chapter 5 on hypertension), not only relieve symptoms of heart failure but also prolong the life of the victims of advanced heart failure.

### Avoiding Sodium Retention

Because retention of sodium, chloride, and water is so important in the manifestations of heart failure, major attention is paid to this part of the problem. It is important to reduce the intake of sodium chloride, and that can only be done by adjusting diet. Avoiding the use of a saltshaker will usually reduce sodium and chloride intake by about one-third. To reduce salt intake further, it is necessary to change the way one prepares food. Many prepackaged foods are rich in salt, and the salt is "hidden." One has to become a label reader. See page 180 for a list of foods that often contribute to an excess intake of sodium.

## Use Diuretics Sparingly

Diuretics, described in chapter 5 in the treatment of hypertension, are a mainstay in the treatment of heart failure. One might ask, If diuretics are so effective in removing sodium and chloride from the body, why bother with diet? The answer is that the more salt one eats, the greater the demand one makes of a diuretic. The greater the dose that one has to use, the more likely that complications of diuretic use will occur. One common and important manifestation of high-dose diuretic use is the loss of potassium and magnesium from the body—a loss that may not be replaced easily and may be dangerous. Many physicians routinely prescribe a diuretic combination that provides some potassium-sparing action for people who also take digitalis but that is sometimes only relatively effective. A deficit of potassium makes digitalis a more dangerous drug.

---

### CUTTING DOWN ON SODIUM

Make it a habit to check labels for sodium content.

Experiment with using lemon juice or vinegar when you cook—they can mimic a "salt" taste.

At restaurants, stick with food at its freshest and most natural. Stay away from sauces.

The American Heart Association furnishes this tip in its publication *Cooking Without Your Salt Shaker*:

> Combine one-half teaspoon of cayenne pepper, one tablespoon of garlic powder, and one teaspoon each of the following ground seasonings: basil, marjoram, thyme, parsley, savory, mace, onion powder, black pepper, and sage.
>
> Try this as a substitute for salt.

---

## SODIUM CONTENT OF FOODS

| Food | Amount | Sodium (milligrams) | Food | Amount | Sodium (milligrams) |
|---|---|---|---|---|---|
| A.1.® Sauce | 1 tbs. | 278 | Quarter Pounder® | 1 | 735 |
| Accent® | 1 tsp. | 518 | Quarter Pounder® | | |
| Anchovy paste | 1 tbs. | 1540 | with cheese | 1 | 1236 |
| Bacon | 1 slice | 209 | Strawberry | | |
| Baking soda | 1 tsp. | 1200 | sundae | 1 | 96 |
| Baking powder | 1 tsp. | 400 | Arby's® | | |
| Barbecue sauce | 1/2 cup | 1019 | Roast beef | 1 | 880 |
| Beans, dried, no salt | 1 cup | 13 | Super roast beef | 1 | 1420 |
| Beef bouillon | 1 cube | 960 | Turkey deluxe | 1 | 1220 |
| Bisquick® | 1 cup | 1475 | Club sandwich | 1 | 1610 |
| Broccoli, frozen in | | | Dairy Queen® | | |
| cheese sauce | 1/2 cup | 331 | Brazier® chili dog | 1 | 939 |
| Catsup | 1 tbs. | 177 | Super Brazier® | | |
| Cabbage, fresh | | | dog | 1 | 1552 |
| shredded | 1/2 cup | 7 | Frozen dinners (ap- | | |
| Celery | 1 stalk | 50 | proximate values) | | |
| Celery seasoning | 1 tsp. | 1430 | beef chop suey | | |
| Cereal | | | with rice | 12 oz. | 2040 |
| cornflakes | 1 cup | 251 | beef pie | 10 oz. | 1600 |
| oatmeal | | | broccoli au gratin | 10 oz. | 470 |
| regular, no salt | 3/4 cup | trace | chicken crepes with | | |
| instant | 3/4 cup | 255 | mushroom sauce | 8 oz. | 1040 |
| shredded wheat | 1 cup | 2 | chicken pie | 10 oz. | 1530 |
| Cheese | | | corn soufflé | 12 oz. | 510 |
| cheddar | 1/2 cup | 350 | green bean mush- | | |
| cottage (2% fat) | 1/2 cup | 459 | room casserole | 9.5 oz. | 1350 |
| processed | 1/2 cup | 812 | green pepper steak | | |
| Cheese soufflé, | | | with rice | 10 oz. | 1500 |
| homemade | 1 cup | 346 | ham and asparagus | | |
| Cherries, raw | 1 cup | 2 | crepes | 6 oz. | 840 |
| Cherry pie | 1/6 of 9" | 480 | pizza, cheese | 10.5 oz. | 850 |
| Chicken, no skin | 2 pieces | 32 | pizza, sausage | 12 oz. | 1320 |
| Chili, canned | 1 cup | 1354 | pot pie | 1 | 1807 |
| Chili sauce | 1 tbs. | 200 | spaghetti with meat | | |
| Chocolate, baking | 100 grams | 3 | sauce | 14 oz. | 1970 |
| Chocolate fudge top- | | | tuna noodle | | |
| ping (Hershey's®) | 100 grams | 115 | casserole | 11.5 oz. | 670 |
| Cocoa mix | | | Fruit, fresh | 1/2 cup | 0 |
| (Hershey's®) | 100 grams | 505 | Fruit pie, Hostess® | 1 | 605 |
| Dill pickle | 1 | 928 | Garlic salt | 1 tsp. | 1850 |
| Fast foods | | | Lemon juice | 1 tbs. | trace |
| McDonald's® | | | Macaroni and | | |
| Egg McMuffin® | 1 | 885 | cheese, packaged | 1 cup | 574–1086 |
| Big Mac® | 1 | 1010 | Margarine, Nucoa® | 1 tbs. | 160 |
| Hamburger | 1 | 520 | Margarine, Mazola® | 1 tbs. | 115 |

## SODIUM CONTENT OF FOODS (continued)

| Food | Amount | Sodium (milligrams) | Food | Amount | Sodium (milligrams) |
|------|--------|--------------------|------|--------|--------------------|
| Margarine, diet | | | Ravioli, canned | 1 cup | 1349 |
| Mazola® | 1 tbs. | 135 | Salad dressing, | | |
| Mayonnaise | 1 tbs. | 84 | bottled | 1 tbs. | 200 |
| Meats, processed | | | Salt | 1 tsp. | 2132 |
| bologna | 1 oz. | 369 | Salt, Morton Lite® | 1 tsp. | 1188 |
| chipped beef | 1/2 cup | 3526 | Sardines, drained | 1 oz. | 2093 |
| corned beef | 3 oz. | 802 | Sauerkraut, canned | 1/2 cup | 878 |
| cured ham | 3 oz. | 863 | Soups, commercial | | |
| frankfurters | 2 oz. | 627 | bean and pork | 1 cup | 2136 |
| pepperoni | 1 oz. | 425 | chicken gumbo | 1 cup | 1940 |
| sausage | 1 link | 290 | chicken noodle | 1 cup | 979 |
| turkey ham | 3 oz. | 865 | chicken and rice | 1 cup | 1872 |
| Meat tenderizer | 1 tsp. | 1700 | clam chowder | 1 cup | 1015 |
| Milk | | | cream of | | |
| whole | 1 cup | 227 | asparagus | 1 cup | 984 |
| 2% | 1 cup | 276 | cream of celery | 1 cup | 1950 |
| nonfat | 1 cup | 233 | cream of chicken | 1 cup | 1982 |
| Monosodium gluta- | | | Cup-A-Soup™ | 1 pkg. | 900 |
| mate (MSG) | 1 tsp. | 750 | split pea | 1 cup | 1956 |
| Mustard | 1 tbs. | 150 | turkey noodle | 1 cup | 2038 |
| Olives | 10 | 686 | vegetable beef | 1 cup | 2135 |
| Onion salt | 1 tsp. | 1620 | vegetable with beef | | |
| Orange juice | 1 cup | 0.2 | broth | 1 cup | 1725 |
| Pancake—mix, | | | Soy sauce | 1 tsp. | 440 |
| egg, milk | 1 | 412 | Tortilla chips, | | |
| Peanut butter, | | | Doritos® | 1 oz. | 193 |
| Skippy® | 2 tbs. | 150 | Tomato | | |
| Peanut Butter Cups, | | | raw | 1 cup | 40 |
| Reese's® | 100 grams | 320 | canned | 1 cup | 313 |
| Pickle, dill | 1 small | 800 | juice | 1 cup | 486 |
| Pizza, cheese | 1 piece | 768 | sauce | 1 cup | 1662 |
| Potato, baked, plain | 1 | 6 | Tuna, canned | 1/2 cup | 679 |
| Potato chips, | | | TV dinner | 1 | 1400 |
| Ruffles® | 1 oz. | 364 | V-8® juice | 1 cup | 700 |
| Pudding, instant | | | Worcestershire | | |
| vanilla | 1/2 cup | 406 | sauce | 1 tbs. | 315 |

(Source: Nutritive Value of American Foods in Common Units. Agricultural Handbook 456, USDA, 1975.)

(Source: McDonald's Corporation, Oak Brook, Illinois: Nutritional Analysis by Raltech Services, Inc., Madison, Wisconsin.)

(Source: Consumer Affairs, Arby's Inc., Atlanta, Georgia: Nutritional Analysis by Technological Resources, Camden, New Jersey.)

(Source: International Dairy Queen Inc., Minneapolis, Minn. Nutritional Analysis by Raltech Services Inc., Madison, Wisconsin.)

## WHAT'S IN OUR FAST FOOD

| | Calories | Protein (grams) | Fat (grams) | Sodium (milligrams) |
|---|---|---|---|---|
| **Arby's®** | | | | |
| Regular roast beef sandwich | 353 | 22.2 | 14.8 | 588 |
| Philly Beef 'N Swiss® | 460 | 24.4 | 28.4 | 1,300 |
| Beef 'N Cheddar® | 455 | 25.7 | 26.8 | 955 |
| Chicken breast sandwich | 509 | 25.9 | 29.1 | 1,082 |
| French fries | 215 | 2.1 | 9.7 | 114 |
| Vanilla shake | 330 | 10.5 | 11.5 | 281 |
| **McDonald's®** | | | | |
| Hamburger | 263 | 12.4 | 11.3 | 510 |
| Cheeseburger | 318 | 15 | 16 | 740 |
| Quarter Pounder® | 427 | 24.6 | 23.5 | 720 |
| Big Mac® | 570 | 24.6 | 35 | 980 |
| Filet-O-Fish® | 435 | 14.7 | 25.7 | 800 |
| McNuggets® | 323 | 19.1 | 20.2 | 510 |
| Egg McMuffin® | 340 | 18.5 | 15.8 | 885 |
| French fries | 220 | 3 | 11.5 | 110 |
| Vanilla shake | 352 | 9.3 | 8.4 | 200 |
| **Church's®** | | | | |
| Chicken breast | 278 | 21.3 | 17.3 | 560 |
| Thigh | 305.8 | 18.5 | 21.6 | 448 |
| Leg | 147 | 12.9 | 8.6 | 286 |
| French fries | 138 | 2.1 | 5.5 | 126 |
| **Popeyes®** | | | | |
| Chicken breast | 428 | 33 | 26 | 876 |
| Wing | 185 | 10 | 13 | 346 |
| Cajun rice | 177 | 9 | 6 | 391 |
| Red beans, small order | 330 | 8 | 19 | 675 |
| Biscuit | 261 | 3 | 16 | 463 |
| **Burger King®** | | | | |
| Whopper® | 628 | 27 | 36 | 880 |
| Hamburger | 275 | 15 | 12 | 509 |
| Bacon double cheeseburger | 510 | 33 | 31 | 728 |
| Chicken sandwich | 688 | 26 | 40 | 1,423 |
| Whaler® | 488 | 19 | 27 | 592 |
| Onion rings | 275 | 4 | 16 | 665 |
| Vanilla shake | 321 | 9 | 10 | 205 |
| **Taco Bell®** | | | | |
| Beef burrito | 402 | 21.7 | 17.3 | 993.9 |
| Beef tostada | 322 | 15.0 | 19.59 | 764 |
| Taco | 183.9 | 10.17 | 10.948 | 273.49 |
| Taco salad | 949.4 | 36.071 | 62.136 | 1,763.1 |

## SEEKING THE IMMEDIATE CAUSE
## OF HEART FAILURE

Once therapy has been instituted, the physician will search for treatable causes of the heart failure. The possible contribution of high blood pressure, anemia, and a hyperactive thyroid gland have already been mentioned. Those with an already damaged heart may have an episode of heart failure because they have taken something that depresses the heart. Examples include an excessive amount of alcohol, and beta-adrenergic blocking agents used for the treatment of high blood pressure. Other examples are some of the drugs used for treating cancer (for example, adriamycin) and some of the drugs used for treating cardiac arrhythmias (disopyramide, for example). Some widely used agents such as cortisone, estrogens, and nonsteroidal anti-inflammatory agents used for treating pain (such as ibuprofen) may cause salt (sodium chloride) and water retention, which in turn can aggravate heart failure. This has become a more common problem since ibuprofen became available without a prescription.

The medical evaluation will also attempt to rule out causes that can be corrected by surgery. For example, if one or more heart valves are found to be abnormal, surgical correction or replacement of the valve can produce a dramatic improvement in the function of the heart. Among older individuals, one of the more common correctable problems involves the development of a stiff valve, the aortic valve, between the left ventricle and the aorta. This problem, called calcific aortic stenosis, can be reversed easily by surgery and, more recently, by valvuloplasty (see chapter 4), and a careful examination is made for this problem in any older person who develops heart failure. If coronary artery disease caused the heart failure, coronary bypass surgery or angioplasty can improve the blood flow to the heart, thus making it easier for the heart to do its job.

## DIGITALIS

Among the herbal medicines identified by folklore were extracts of squill (the bulb of the seed onion) and the foxglove. The ancient Egyptians and Chinese over a thousand years ago used squill to treat dropsy, the accumulation of massive amounts of fluid. William Withering introduced to Western society the use of extract of foxglove for the treatment of dropsy over two hundred years ago. The active principle, in each case, was the chemical digitalis. Today, of course, physicians no longer prescribe herbal extracts but rather a synthetic material made by the pharmaceutical industry. The potency and activity of digitalis from lot to lot is obviously much better, and the result is a much more predictable product.

Digitalis has two actions that help the heart. In the person with an irregular and rapid heart action, which can contribute to the poor function of the pump, digitalis slows the response of the left ventricle. Digitalis also acts to improve the contraction of the heart muscle in a heart that has failed, though this action is probably more modest. Today, many physicians continue to debate the contribution of the latter action to the overall performance of the heart, but digitalis remains a standard.

## What to Watch For

The individual taking digitalis (digoxin is the most commonly used preparation) should be aware of several important points. Digitalis can provoke arrhythmias (see chapter 12) and is especially likely to do so in the person who has a low serum potassium and magnesium concentration. Intake of potassium and magnesium may be marginal because of dietary selection (see pages 183–185 for a listing of foods rich in potassium and magnesium). In addition, the common use of thiazide-type diuretics by the person with heart failure, especially in larger doses, promotes the excretion of potassium and magnesium. That can be prevented by the use of a potassium-sparing diuretic combination (triamterene, amiloride, or spironolactone), by potassium supplementation of the diet (though potassium supplements do not restore magnesium), or through the use of a converting enzyme inhibitor (captopril or enalapril).

Many doctors recommend the use of a salt substitute for the individual with heart failure. It is important to recognize that many of the salt substitutes are especially rich in potassium. If you are using a potassium-sparing diuretic, it is possible to have too much potassium in the serum, so you have to combine a potassium supplement with a potassium-sparing diuretic very carefully. This requires the specific advice of your physician.

Digoxin is excreted primarily by the kidneys. If the intake of digoxin is too large, the serum concentration can rise to toxic levels. Because this toxicity can be very important, and even

## SOURCES OF MAGNESIUM

| Food | Serving | Milligrams per Serving |
|---|---|---|
| Almonds | 1/2 cup | 270 |
| Apple | 3-1/4″ diameter | 16 |
| Applesauce, canned, sweetened | 1/2 cup | 5 |
| Brazil nuts | 25 | 225 |
| Bread | | |
| pumpernickel | 1 slice | 23 |
| whole wheat | 1 slice | 18 |
| Carrots and peas, frozen, cooked | 1/2 cup | 19 |
| Cashew nuts | 1 cup | 427 |
| Chicken, white meat, stewed | 3–4 ounces | 19 |
| Coffee | 1 cup, black | 21.8 |
| Graham crackers | 7 | 51 |
| Hamburger, lean, broiled | 3–4 ounces | 25 |
| Milk | | |
| chocolate | 1/2 cup | 58 |
| skim | 1/2 cup | 14 |
| whole | 1/2 cup | 13 |
| Orange, sections without membrane | 1/2 cup | 13 |
| Peach, fresh | 2-1/2″ diameter | 8 |
| Peanut butter | 6 tablespoons | 30 |
| Peanuts, roasted, shelled | 1 cup | 280 |
| Prune juice, canned or bottled, unsweetened | 3 ounces | 10 |
| Rice | | |
| brown, cooked | 1/2 cup | 29 |
| white, cooked | 1/2 cup | 8 |
| Shredded wheat cereal | 4 large biscuits or 2 cups spoon-sized biscuits | 133 |
| Spinach, fresh, chopped | 2 cups | 88 |
| Tomato, fresh | 2-3/5″ diameter | 11 |
| Tomato soup, canned, condensed, diluted to serve | 1/2 cup | 9 |
| Walnuts, broken | 4/5 cup | 134 |

**SODIUM AND POTASSIUM CONTENT OF FRUITS AND VEGETABLES**

| Food | Serving Size | Potassium per Serving (milligrams) | Sodium per Serving (milligrams) | Calories |
|---|---|---|---|---|
| Apple juice | 1 cup | 250 | 2 | 117 |
| Avocado | 1 half | 650 | 5 | 185 |
| Banana | 1 medium | 500 | 1 | 127 |
| Blackberries | 1 cup | 245 | 1 | 84 |
| Broccoli | 1 cup cooked | 414 | 16 | 40 |
| Brussels sprouts | 1 cup cooked | 423 | 16 | 56 |
| Cantaloupe | 1 cup cubes | 400 | 19 | 40 |
| Grapefruit juice | 1 cup, canned | 405 | 2 | 135 |
| Honeydew melon | 1 cup cubes | 374 | 20 | 50 |
| Lima beans | 1 cup cooked | 1,163 | 4 | 262 |
| Orange | 1 medium | 263 | 1 | 65 |
| Orange juice | 1 cup | 496 | 2 | 110 |
| Peach | 1 medium | 202 | 1 | 38 |
| Pear | 1 medium | 260 | 4 | 122 |
| Potato | 1 large, baked in skin | 782 | 6 | 145 |
| Prune juice | 1 cup | 602 | 5 | 195 |
| Prunes | 10 medium | 310 | 5 | 110 |
| Rutabaga | 1 cup cooked | 284 | 7 | 60 |
| Spinach | 1 cup raw | 259 | 39 | 14 |
| Split peas | 1 cup cooked | 592 | 26 | 230 |
| Tomato | 1 medium | 366 | 4 | 33 |
| Watermelon | 1 cup cubes | 100 | 1 | 26 |
| White beans | 1 cup cooked | 790 | 13 | 224 |

life-threatening, it is important to recognize the early warning signals of digitalis overdose, which are the same whatever preparation is being taken. Loss of appetite, nausea, and vomiting are the most common early symptoms of digitalis overdose. Diarrhea, abdominal pain, and bloating can also occur. That does not mean, of course, that all individuals on digitalis who lose their appetite and become nauseated and vomit have digitalis overdose; intestinal flu is a common cause of all three symptoms. On the other hand, the appearance of such symptoms suggests that a call to one's physician is in order. The problem of differentiating digitalis intoxication from flu is compounded by

## SOURCES OF POTASSIUM

| Food | Serving | Milligrams per Serving |
|---|---|---|
| Almonds, chopped | 1/2 cup | 500 |
| Apricots, dried, uncooked | 3/4 cup | 954 |
| Banana | 1 medium | 500 |
| Beets, diced, cooked | 1/2 cup | 140 |
| Broccoli, chopped | 1/2 cup | 190 |
| Brussels sprouts | 2/3 cup | 305 |
| Cantaloupe | 1/8 | 170 |
| Carrots, raw, grated | 1 cup | 375 |
| Celery, raw, diced | 1 cup | 409 |
| Chicken, broiled, bones removed | 3 ounces | 245 |
| Chili con carne with beans, canned | 1/2 cup | 290 |
| Cocoa | 1 cup | 210 |
| Eggs, hard boiled | 2 | 130 |
| Flounder | 4 ounces | 375 |
| Halibut | 4 ounces | 500 |
| Milk | | |
| whole | 1/2 cup | 150 |
| 2% | 1/2 cup | 170 |
| Mushrooms, raw, sliced | 1 cup | 290 |
| Peaches, dried, uncooked | 1/2 cup | 525 |
| Potato, dehydrated flakes (water, milk, butter, and salt added ) | 1/2 cup | 300 |
| Potato, white, baked, skin removed | 1 | 500 |
| Prune juice, canned or bottled | 1/2 cup | 300 |
| Spaghetti, enriched, with meatballs and tomato sauce | | |
| home recipe | 1/2 cup | 330 |
| canned | 1/2 cup | 120 |
| Sugar, brown, tightly packed | 1 cup | 757 |
| Sunflower seeds, dry, hulled | 1 cup | 1,334 |
| Walnuts, English, chopped | 1 cup | 540 |

the fact that occasionally digitalis intoxication will cause diarrhea. Headache is relatively common, as is visual blurring.

One unusual form of visual change in the person suffering from digitalis intoxication involves color vision. Objects are described as having a yellow or green halo around them.

Finally, there are disturbances of the heart's rhythm that might be recognized as palpitations by the person who has taken too much digitalis.

The development of very precise and accurate methods for measuring the concentration of digoxin in serum has simplified judgments about adjusting digitalis dosage. This technical advance has made the use of digitalis much safer over the past ten years.

## General Digoxin

Generic forms of digoxin are available. A widely cited study performed over a decade ago showed that the generic digoxin compounds available then were much more variable in their potency, and much less predictable in their utility, than was the agent produced under a trade name. This study led to an important improvement in the quality control of generic agents. Today, there is no reason to believe that the generic digoxin differs in any substantive way from those sold with a trade name.

## DIURETICS

There are two broad categories of diuretic agents, the thiazide-type diuretics (see chapter 5) and the loop diuretics. Loop diuretics are used substantially less often in the treatment of high blood pressure, unless the individual being treated has abnormally reduced kidney function, but they are very important to the individual with heart failure.

## Loop Diuretics

Loop diuretics, such as furosemide, ethacrynic acid, and bumetanide, work on a different part of the kidney than do the thiazides. As a consequence, they are much more potent and can produce a much larger loss of sodium, chloride, and water. They tend to work very quickly and produce a very large response, so it is important to select a convenient time for taking them. Because they are likely to result in trips to the bathroom to empty the bladder every forty to sixty minutes for as long as several hours, obviously bedtime is a poor time to take a loop diuretic! Just prior to departure on a bus or a car trip is an equally poor time. People who take a loop diuretic typically discover their pattern of response and individualize the most appropriate time for taking the medication.

### Side Effects of Loop Diuretics

As was the case with thiazide diuretics, loop diuretics can result in critically important losses of potassium and magnesium. The same warnings apply, though no convenient potassium-sparing loop diuretic is currently available. If a loop diuretic is used, careful attention to details of diet to maximize potassium and magnesium intake relative to sodium intake is important (see pages 183–185).

One problem with the loop diuretics can be their potency. It is possible to overtreat with them so that sodium, chloride, and water are depleted. The result is equivalent to dehydration, and the major impact is on kidney function. The individual most prone to develop this side effect is the one who takes the loop diuretic faithfully in spite of intestinal flu—with its symptoms of appetite loss, nausea, vomiting, and diarrhea. The problem is particularly important if the person is also taking digitalis because the reduction in kidney function produced by the dehydration can increase the digitalis concentration in serum dramatically.

Omitting doses of the loop diuretic is a good idea when vomiting and diarrhea are a problem. It is an equally good idea to contact one's physician at the same time. A visit to the doctor's office, which ordinarily might not be undertaken for a mild case of flu, is often a very good idea for the person who has had heart failure and who is being treated with digitalis and a loop diuretic.

Generic versions of the most widely used drugs (furosemide and ethacrynic acid) are available.

## CAPTOPRIL AND ENALAPRIL

The role of the renin-angiotensin-aldosterone system in the function in the body of sodium and chloride was reviewed in chapter 2. Because heart failure results in the edema reflecting retention of both along with water, it is not surprising that the renin-angiotensin system plays a role in the heart failure story. Converting enzyme inhibitors that work by virtue of their ability to block formation of angiotensin II quickly found a place in the treatment of heart failure. Indeed, they are the only drugs among the vasodilators currently approved by the FDA for heart failure treatment.

Converting enzyme inhibitors improve heart failure in several ways. First, by dilating the small arteries, they reduce the work of the heart. Second, by dilating the arteries to the kidneys, and thus improving blood flow, they facilitate the kidneys' ability to handle sodium. Third, by blocking production of aldosterone, they not only improve excretion of sodium but also reduce the unhealthy loss of potassium and magnesium that occurs when aldosterone levels are high.

Finally, by dilating veins, converting enzyme inhibitors shift blood away from the lungs, reducing the fluid in the lungs and shortness of breath. Studies have shown that these drugs improve the function of the cardiovascular system and the kidneys and the exercise tolerance of individuals with heart failure.

The side effects of converting enzyme inhibitors were discussed in chapter 5, when the treatment of high blood pressure was reviewed. The only difference in side effects when the problem is heart failure is that blood pressure may not be as high before treatment, so a fall in blood pressure resulting in dizziness may be somewhat more frequent. Although this dizziness has often led to discontinuation of the use of a converting enzyme inhibitor, that may be a mistake. There is evidence that such an agent is likely to be especially effective. A much better solution is to reduce the dose by breaking up the tablets. That also has the virtue of reducing the cost substantially!

No generic forms of a converting enzyme inhibitor are available or will be in the near future.

### Converting Enzyme Inhibitors as Prevention?

It is possible that converting enzyme inhibitors are beneficial in even more ways than described earlier. In animal models, treatment with a converting enzyme inhibitor has changed the progression of the disease. For reasons that are not yet entirely clear, treatment with such agents, and not with other vasodilators, prevents the change in heart structure that leads to further heart failure. Clinical trials in people with heart disease are now under way to see whether the same principle applies.

If the goal of treatment is to relieve severe symptoms, clearly treatment should not be undertaken until those severe symptoms occur. That is, one should delay treatment with captopril until it is mandated by symptoms not controlled well by diet, digitalis, and loop diuretics. On the other hand, if captopril and other converting enzyme inhibitors prevent the progression of heart disease, a compelling argument exists to begin treatment much earlier, at the first sign that heart disease is present and might be progressive. During the next several years, researchers should have the answer to the fundamental question of *when* to start treatment with a converting enzyme inhibitor.

## PROGRESS IN THE FIGHT AGAINST HEART FAILURE

The past two decades have seen progressive and dramatic improvement in physicians' ability to treat virtually everyone who develops heart failure. In some cases, identification of a specific problem has led to what earlier would have been considered a miraculous improvement. Control of high blood pressure has sharply reduced the frequency of heart failure, since this was once among the most common causes. Doctors can already anticipate an equivalent reduction in the frequency and severity of heart failure with the new treatments for myocardial infarction. Reduction of risk factors should decrease further the frequency of myocardial infarction.

Eventually, however, these treatments become inadequate for at least some individuals. In the past few years, a number of heart transplants have been done, and assist devices designed to maintain at least partial heart function while a heart transplant can be sought have been implanted. One of the more dramatic recent announcements involved the modification of skeletal muscle in the back by a surgical technique and electrical stimulation so that it can fill at least part of the function of the left ventricle. That is clearly still a research procedure, but it holds real promise.

Prevention is clearly better than even the dramatic improvements in treatment. Fortunately, doctors can prevent rheumatic heart disease with antibiotics for streptococcal disease, effective use of antihypertensive agents can prevent hypertension-induced heart failure, the new treatments of coronary artery thrombosis are likely to reduce muscle damage from atherosclerosis, and careful attention to lifestyle will reduce the frequency and severity of coronary artery disease. The old saying "An ounce of prevention . . ." certainly applies here.

# 12

# Arrhythmias

For the heart to function as a pump, the millions of muscle cells that make up the heart have to contract together, in a synchronized manner. For each contraction, all these cells must pull together and then stop pulling, simultaneously, so that the heart can relax and fill with blood. To accomplish this, a specialized area in the heart, called the pacemaker, spontaneously sends out an electrical signal that is rapidly spread throughout the heart and leads to contraction. The heart rate is increased when we are physically active and decreased when we are resting or asleep through the actions of nerves and hormones on that pacemaker.

Because this system results in a regular, normal heart rhythm, abnormalities in the system lead to what is commonly known as arrhythmias.

A large variety of arrhythmias of the heart exist, and the most common is the most benign. Many individuals have occasional irregular beats of which they are unaware and that become apparent only when the heart or pulse is being examined or during an electrocardiogram.

## TYPES OF ARRHYTHMIA

It is useful to divide arrhythmias into those that result in a very rapid rate of heart action, the tachycardias, and those that result in too slow a heart action, the bradycardias. In some cases, the heart rate remains in the normal range, from 60 to 100 beats per minute, but there is an irregularity in that beat.

The individual with an irregular heart action is typically unaware of it. By far the most common form of arrhythmia is known as a premature beat, which, in the absence of heart disease, is not important. The irregular beats appear in isolated fashion at infrequent intervals and produce either a minimal, momentary awareness or no symptoms at all. Without associated heart disease, these premature beats do not influence longevity or suitability for life insurance, military service, or employment.

## Palpitations

The word *palpitations* indicates heartbeats that have come to an individual's attention. In the case of the premature beat, persons occasionally notice a thump in their chest that reflects not the premature beat but the next beat. Because a premature beat occurs early, there is often a compensatory pause, and the next beat is larger than normal—larger because, with that pause, the heart has more time to fill with blood, and thus a larger heartbeat with the ejection of more blood follows. The person feels that larger beat as an accentuated contraction.

Premature beats generally do not require treatment, and drug treatment is rarely required. In some cases, they are clearly provoked or made more frequent by use of coffee, tea, or caffeine-containing soft drinks; cigarettes; or alcohol. There are many reasons for limiting alcohol use and eliminating smoking in any case.

When an individual is taking diuretic drugs, the presence of premature beats may reflect abnormalities of electrolytes (see chapter 5), bringing on the arrhythmia. In that case, an adjustment of the diuretic used or of the diet may be necessary to correct the electrolyte abnormality (see chapter 11 for sources of potassium and magnesium).

## IMPACT OF A SLOW HEART RATE

When the heart rate is too slow, there is often a real impact on how the body functions. When heart rate falls to low levels, the output of blood from the heart—the cardiac output required to provide blood flow to all the organs—is limited. The fall in blood pressure and cardiac output often affects the nervous system. If the heart rate suddenly falls to a very low level, the individual may suddenly lose consciousness. Because this loss of consciousness (called Stokes-Adams syndrome) resembles fainting, close attention is paid to the heart when someone faints without apparent reason.

For older persons, especially, a prolonged period of low cardiac output can express itself as confusion. Correction of the very slow heart rate can promote a striking improvement in clarity of thinking. Some people who already have an abnormal heart experience very low heart rate as shortness of breath, which is actually a reflection of heart failure (see chapter 11). When someone has coronary artery disease, the very low cardiac output can promote chest pain.

## PACING THE HEART

In the short run, drugs that block the action of the vagus nerve (see figure 23) on the pacemaker area, such as atropine sulfate, may be used to increase heart rate. The action of the vagus

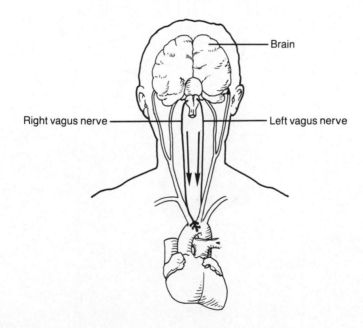

**Figure 23.    The Vagus Nerve**
The vagus nerve runs from the brain to the heart. When this nerve is activated, the result is a strong slowing of the heart. That can occur, for example, during a fainting episode. When the heart beats too slowly, drugs that block the action of the vagus nerve can be used to increase the heart rate.

nerve on the pacemaker tends to slow the heart. In the long run, these drugs tend to have too many side effects for continued use, so it is often best to employ an external cardiac pacemaker (see figure 24). The pacing system consists of a device that generates electrical stimuli for delivery to the heart through electrodes (electrical leads) placed on the heart. The electrodes may be used temporarily, when reversible factors are present, or can be implanted permanently.

A variety of pacing systems are available. They differ according to how the leads are placed (through the venous system without opening the chest; or by a surgical procedure, in which the electrodes are placed directly in the heart), where they are placed, the type of pulse generated, and whether a "sensing system" is used. "Demand" pacemakers have now been

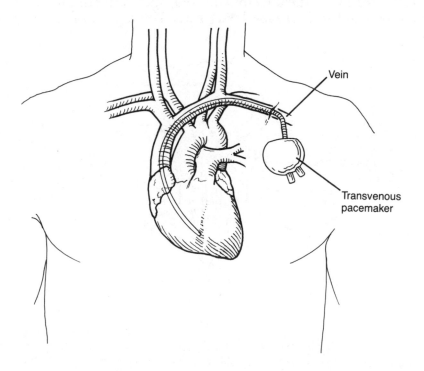

**Figure 24.    A Transvenous Pacemaker**

It is possible to place a pacemaker to control the heartbeat rate and its regularity without opening the chest. In the example shown, the electrodes have been placed through a vein in the arm. In other cases, the electrodes are placed directly on the heart, and the control system is placed under the skin (not shown).

developed that will come into play only when they are needed. These require a sensing system to recognize that they are needed. Others operate continuously. Because the electrical energy comes from a battery, the effectiveness of the battery has to be monitored regularly. Development of electronic pacemakers has improved the quality and the length of many people's lives.

### When to Use an Electronic Pacemaker

When a person has lost consciousness without apparent reason several times, the decision to use an electronic pacemaker is easy for the doctor. In other cases, judgment is involved. When a physician suggests that an electronic pacemaker be used, it is reasonable to ask why the pacemaker is required, what the expectations of benefit are, and what other options are available. If the answers to these questions leave you in doubt, it is reasonable to request a second opinion.

## IMPACT OF A FAST HEART RATE

Tachycardias generally lead to disagreeable palpitations and an awareness of a rapid heart action. Because a heart beating very rapidly cannot provide adequate blood flow, fatigue and breathlessness often occur. As in the case of the bradycardias, the tachycardias vary widely in their mechanism and in the approaches to treatment. They may be sustained or intermittent and can be considered an emergency requiring immediate and prolonged treatment or an episode that, once treated, is unlikely to recur.

## ALTERNATIVE APPROACHES TO TREATMENT OF ARRHYTHMIAS

Aside from the measures described above, a wide variety of drugs and of alternative approaches to treatment are available. Alternatives include cardioversion, which converts arrhythmias to normal rhythm by the application of a direct electrical current to the heart. Developed over twenty years ago, this is now a widely used method for treatment of emergencies as well as an elective treatment of rapid or irregular heart action. Cardioversion is less likely to be used when it is believed that the arrhythmia will recur immediately or when attempts at cardioversion may lead to more serious arrhythmias.

Occasionally, surgery may be helpful for the treatment of arrhythmias that have not responded well to drug therapy or pacemakers.

## EVALUATING ARRHYTHMIAS

A number of sophisticated approaches to the evaluation of arrhythmias have been developed. In one category of evaluation, the Holter monitor is used. The individual wears an apparatus with electrodes placed on his or her chest and elsewhere on the body so that the rhythm of the heart can be assessed in the course of normal daily activity (see chapter 4). This approach permits analysis of arrhythmia frequency and complexity; correlation with an individual's symptoms; and evaluation of the effect of antiarrhythmic therapy, especially drug therapy.

As an alternative, an invasive procedure may be used. Specialized catheters containing electrodes may be placed in various positions within the heart to record electrical activity at specific locations. The information might be used to improve on drug therapy or to help in making a decision about whether surgery might be helpful by cutting an area that leads to arrhythmias. Indeed, these catheters have been used to cut or cauterize an offending area, thereby treating the arrhythmia. This approach might also be used to test the effect of various drugs.

## DRUGS THAT REGULATE
## THE HEART'S RHYTHM

Details in the use of the available antiarrhythmic drugs are important, for two reasons. First, the difference between the dose required to achieve the desired effect and the dose likely to be toxic is often rather slight. Second, the aim of treatment is to maintain an adequate level of the drug in the body tissues with the minimum possible fluctuation. For each drug, the dose must be carefully defined to minimize toxicity and maximize the impact on the arrhythmia.

Another feature of the antiarrhythmic drugs is that they can also actually *provoke* arrhythmias, which can make for a complex situation. The physician must sometimes untangle the primary arrhythmia from the drug-provoked arrhythmia. Also, many of the drugs have a tendency to reduce the ability of the heart to pump blood, so in a case of borderline heart function, heart failure can be precipitated. Since the arrhythmias themselves can cause heart failure, once again the situation is complicated.

## Digitalis

Digitalis strengthens the heart's contractions (see chapter 11), but it also has an important role in treating arrhythmias. The side effects of digitalis often involve the gastrointestinal tract (loss of appetite, nausea, vomiting, diarrhea, abdominal pain, and bloating). Toxic side effects involving the central nervous system include fatigue and weakness, psychological disturbances, and a change in color vision (objects might develop a yellow or green characteristic).

## Quinidine

Quinidine sulfate has been used in the treatment of some arrhythmias for many years. If you are taking digitalis and your doctor suggests that you also take quinidine, it is important to point out that you are already taking digitalis, since the combination can raise the amount of digoxin in the body substantially. Adverse effects of quinidine involve the gastrointestinal tract (nausea, vomiting, and diarrhea) and the central nervous system (a ringing in the ears, hearing impairment, dizziness, double vision, confusion, and headache). The side effects resemble somewhat those induced by digitalis.

## Procainamide

Procainamide hydrochloride has also been used for many years for arrhythmias. Adverse effects involve the gastrointestinal system (loss of appetite, nausea, and vomiting) and the central nervous system (as with the agents above). Some individuals develop a side effect that includes fever, joint aches, and chest pain, reflecting inflammation of the outer lining of the heart.

## Phenytoin

Phenytoin is most widely used as an anticonvulsant drug but also has been employed for cardiac arrhythmias. Adverse side effects are primarily confined to the central nervous system and include drowsiness, rapid eye movements, dizziness, and difficulty in maintaining balance. It is important to review the other drugs being employed when phenytoin is suggested, since it has important interactions with a wide variety of drugs.

### Propranolol

Propranolol, a beta-adrenergic blocking agent, slows the heart rate and is useful for a wide variety of arrhythmias. This drug and its side effects are described in chapter 5.

### Verapamil

Verapamil is a calcium channel blocking agent, widely used for the treatment of angina pectoris and high blood pressure (see chapters 5 and 9). The major adverse reactions to verapamil include too large a fall in blood pressure and constipation.

## PROSPECTS IN THE TREATMENT
## OF ARRHYTHMIAS

Because digitalis, quinidine, procainamide, phenytoin, propranolol, and verapamil have all been used for a long time, generic equivalents are available. This reduces the cost of medication substantially. Unfortunately, for many individuals these drugs are ineffective. A host of newer drugs have been developed, however; many are still not yet approved by the FDA for routine treatment but will be available in the near future. Their use is generally reserved for individuals for whom the earlier agents have been found to be ineffective.

The ability to control cardiac arrhythmias through the use of electrical regulation, surgery, and an increasing number of effective drugs has improved substantially in the past decade. It is important to remember that the most common irregular heart action, the premature beat, has little implication for well-being in the absence of heart disease and does not require treatment. Perhaps the biggest problem in this area is the widespread use of antiarrhythmic drugs in the treatment of persons who actually do not require treatment.

# 13

❧❧❧

# Fainting, Dizziness, and Drop Spells

Scarcely an eight-hour shift goes by in the average hospital emergency room when someone does not appear who has suffered a brief loss of consciousness that cannot be explained immediately. Because dizziness or vertigo often precedes a loss of consciousness, and may be difficult to separate from a partial loss of consciousness, those symptoms will also be discussed in this chapter.

## FAINTING

A simple episode of fainting, which the physician might call a vasovagal attack or syncope, is much the most common cause of unconsciousness, reflecting a fall in blood pressure that occurs because the blood vessels dilate and the heart rate slows. Fainting has no implications for long-term well-being provided no injury occurs when the person falls. Indeed, the fall typically corrects the problem, since it improves the return of blood to the heart from the veins and restores blood pressure.

Because it is so common, and frightening, fainting merits a little more description. There is typically a little warning, an experience of apprehension and anxiety, often associated with palpitations (see chapter 12); giddiness; a peculiar feeling in the abdomen that many describe as "a sinking feeling"; nausea; and a gradual feeling of faintness. Even with complete loss of consciousness, loss of control of bladder or bowel function is extremely rare.

Typically, the attack is self-limited and begins to reverse within moments of lying down, though people will often feel unsteady and unwell for some time afterward. A cold sweat is another typical feature.

Anyone who has seen soldiers on a parade square knows that even the superbly fit, well-conditioned young man or woman can faint. Indeed, soldiers are taught early in their training to flex the muscles in their legs and buttocks periodically when standing and to stand on their toes to prevent such an episode. These maneuvers prevent the pooling of blood in the veins of the legs caused by prolonged standing, especially in the heat.

The treatment of fainting involves lying down. This is a situation in which it is better to lose one's dignity, and lie down, than to try to "fight it out." Indeed, should an episode occur in a confined space, such as a telephone booth, it is important to move the person to a place where he or she can lie down as quickly as possible. Blood flow to the brain falls with the fall in blood pressure, and it is urgent to restore blood pressure and blood flow to the brain by lying down.

## Special Causes

Among individuals older than forty, more complex and important causes of fainting increase in frequency, but even among older individuals the problem is benign more than two-thirds of the time.

The causes of fainting due to an abnormality of the heart were reviewed in chapter 12. Typically, an arrhythmia is responsible. Evaluation will often require obtaining an electrocardiogram and frequently Holter monitoring, which demands wearing an apparatus for continuous electrocardiogram recording for twenty-four hours or more. When suggested by the physician, it is well worth pursuing because the fainting episode can be the first sign of a heart problem that requires treatment.

Brief losses of consciousness due to an abnormality in the nervous system are uncommon but do occur. What appears to

A simple episode of fainting is not a sign of ill health. It is caused by a fall in blood pressure. The treatment is lying down, which speeds the return of blood to the heart.

be a faint can be the first sign of epileptic seizures. Again, a physician is required to identify the seizure with special tests, but clues can be found in the fact that the loss of consciousness does not reverse rapidly when the individual lies down. Loss of bladder or bowel function is also much more common with a seizure.

## What May Provoke a Faint

Fainting may occur for a variety of reasons:

### Drugs

Individuals taking drugs that influence the sympathetic nervous system are more prone to develop a drop in blood pressure when they stand. If the drop in blood pressure is sufficiently large, fainting may occur. The drugs include agents used for the treatment of high blood pressure, such as methyldopa, guanethidine, reserpine, and the alpha-adrenergic blocking agents prazosin, terazosin, and trimazosin as well as antihistamines and many medications used for the treatment of psychiatric illness. In older people, especially after a meal or when first standing, the impact of these drugs is likely to be more substantial.

### Alcohol

Alcohol also dilates blood vessels and can provoke a drop in blood pressure and fainting. This is especially likely to be a problem on a hot day or when drugs that also precipitate fainting are used. (Ask your pharmacist whether alcohol will have any effect on the drugs you may be taking.) Under those circumstances, alcohol-containing beverages should be used judiciously.

### Hyperventilation

An individual who experiences hyperventilation (sustained, rapid, shallow breathing) may have symptoms similar to a fainting episode, though a full loss of consciousness is rare. Hyperventilation most often occurs as part of one's response to anxiety and is associated with sensations of suffocation, a feeling of pressure in the chest, and shortness of breath. Since anxiety provokes the situation, and since the symptoms are also anxiety-provoking, one often gets into a vicious circle. Many of the symptoms are reversed by breathing into a paper bag, which sounds silly but is effective. The reason the paper bag works reflects the fact that hyperventilation causes the loss of a substantial amount of carbon dioxide, and rebreathing from a bag restores the carbon dioxide to the body and reverses many of the symptoms.

### When Fainting Should Send You to Your Doctor

Given the fact that fainting episodes are benign, and much more common than the less benign causes of interruption of consciousness, how should you deal with one? If the episode is absolutely typical, occurs in a setting that might promote fainting (such as prolonged standing, particularly on a hot day), and is associated with transient loss of consciousness that reverses quickly when you lie down, there is little reason for anxiety. If, on the other hand, the attack is not typical, you are taking drugs that might induce a fall in blood pressure, or the loss of consciousness is more prolonged, a visit to your doctor is in order. Fortunately, most of the time the episode is benign, and little more investigation or treatment is required.

## DIZZINESS OR VERTIGO

Body balance is controlled by the nervous system with information from multiple sources, but an especially important part involves the inner ear. If the inner ear sends a signal that is not matched by information from other parts of the body, the individual suffers a feeling of movement in space, often a feeling of spinning, that is called vertigo. Vertigo is frequently accompanied by other symptoms including nausea and vomiting, inability to walk in a coordinated fashion, and falling. Motion sickness, which many have experienced on a boat or in the backseat of a car, is one example. If the inner ear is involved, there may be associated hearing loss or a ringing in the ears.

Fainting never occurs when an individual is lying down. Symptoms of vertigo, on the other hand, are common when a person first lies down in bed at night or when turning over. Should the attack of vertigo occur when you are lying down, or when walking and suddenly turning, it is much more likely to be from the inner ear and not a fainting episode.

## DROP SPELLS

A symptom complex that resembles fainting but does not involve loss of consciousness is a poorly understood phenomenon known as drop spells. The legs of the person suddenly and without warning give way, and the individual falls. Consciousness remains intact, so it is easy to discriminate a drop spell from a fainting episode. For reasons that are unclear, drop spells are much more frequent in women than in men and typically occur in middle age or later.

# 14

# Transient Ischemic Attacks (TIAs) and Stroke

The word *stroke* implies loss of the function of part of the brain because of an interference with its blood supply. Interruption of the blood supply occurs because an artery has become occluded (closed off), due either to a blood clot in an artery damaged by atherosclerosis (see chapter 7) or to a clot that has blocked the vessel by moving through the bloodstream from some other site, typically in the heart or one of the large arteries (see figure 25). Some strokes are due to hemorrhage through a damaged arterial wall, especially in someone with very high blood pressure. The extent of the neuromuscular damage from a stroke depends upon what part of the central nervous system was deprived of its blood supply.

Strokes are common—indeed the most common devastating disease influencing the central nervous system. Their impact can be enormous. Fortunately, the frequency of stroke has been falling progressively over the past two decades, and treatments are now available to prevent or modify the impact of a stroke.

## WARNING OF STROKE—
## A KEY TO PREVENTION

Most strokes give some warning that they might occur. That warning is called a transient ischemic attack, or TIA. A TIA is a temporary episode of dysfunction of the brain due to blockage of a blood vessel. To qualify as a TIA, the episode must resolve completely within twenty-four hours. The majority of TIAs

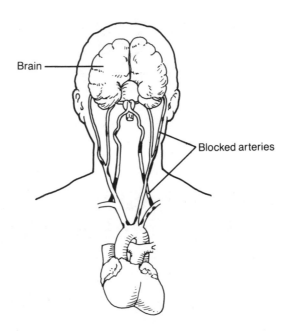

**Figure 25.    Stroke**

A stroke occurs when the arteries to the brain are blocked. Blockage can be due to atherosclerosis, a blood clot that is formed on the area of atherosclerosis, a piece of clot that breaks off and floats through the circulation, or an embolus.

last for two to fifteen minutes. Their importance lies in the fact that they are a marker for stroke. After a TIA, the risk of stroke rises sharply. TIAs typically represent blockage extending from atherosclerosis. The plugs might consist either of aggregates of platelets or of atherosclerotic material, including cholesterol.

## TIA Symptoms

The symptoms of a TIA reflect the blood vessel that has been blocked. One common group of symptoms includes transient loss of vision in one eye, inability to speak, and numbness or weakness on one side involving the face, hand, arm, or leg. Another common grouping includes visual blurring involving both eyes; double vision; vertigo or dizziness; slurred speech; difficulty in swallowing; and difficulty in walking, often with numbness or weakness in an arm or leg. Of course, things other than blood vessel blockage can mimic a transient ischemic attack. In some cases, an X-ray diagnosis is required for the location of the clot.

## Treatment of TIA

Treatment of transient ischemic attack is important. The symptoms must be brought to the attention of a physician. The risk management described earlier for high blood pressure and atherosclerosis is critical. If hypertension is present, it must be treated, and effectively. The same holds true for abnormalities of the heart (such as a cardiac arrhythmia, heart failure, an earlier myocardial infarction that serves as a source for clots, or infection of a heart valve) and hypercholesterolemia. Cigarette smoking must be discontinued.

### Drugs
Direct drug treatment involves the use of aspirin, and other agents that modify platelet function, as in the treatment for angina pectoris (see chapter 9). Anticoagulants to prevent blood clotting are also often used. Recent attempts have been made to use pentoxifylline, a drug developed for treating peripheral arterial disease (see chapter 15) and marketed for that purpose, but that is still a research area.

### Surgical Procedures
A surgical procedure called carotid endarterectomy is sometimes the best choice for an individual having TIAs in whom a blockage of the carotid artery, the large artery in the neck, is identified (see figure 25). There is evidence that successful surgery reduces the likelihood of a subsequent complete stroke.

The extracranial-intracranial bypass operation, a procedure that was widely used prior to 1985, is falling into disfavor because a recent study showed that the bypass surgical procedure failed to prevent stroke or even reduce the occurrence of TIAs.

---

Each year in the United States, approximately 400,000 persons suffer from stroke. It follows heart disease and cancer as a leading cause of death in the nation.

---

## RECOVERY AFTER A STROKE

Seventy-five to 80 percent of the people who suffer a complete stroke survive. Treatment is continued, as described for TIAs, because a substantial number of individuals who suffer a stroke are at risk of another one.

Because swelling of the brain, which today can be visualized easily through the use of CAT scans, tends to make the symptoms worse when they begin, it is not unusual for substantial improvement to occur during the first several days after a stroke. Indeed, return of function of the limbs or speech may continue for months.

Although recovery from a stroke depends primarily on recovery of specific nerves, an active rehabilitation program can help improve functioning. It is important for the individual who has suffered a stroke to find new ways to deal with walking and other activities. Many experts recommend that programs of retraining begin within twenty-four hours of evidence of stability. Rehabilitation programs are available in virtually every area of the country, and physicians will make referrals to them.

The first goals of rehabilitation are to improve the ability to sit, stand, and walk. Walking can begin as soon as the person is able to stand, comfortably, for fifteen to twenty minutes without fatigue. Splints or braces applied to a weak leg can help substantially.

A painful shoulder on the side of a temporarily paralyzed arm is a very common problem for an older person because of a prolonged period of immobility. It may occur despite early passive motion around the shoulder, created by someone else moving the arm. Continued passive movements, combined with heat and occasional cortisone shots, will reduce pain and prevent permanent fixation.

For the individual who has a mild to moderate loss of the ability to speak (dysphasia), speech therapy is often helpful. Speech therapy should involve the family, as family members can be a very helpful encouragement to keep talking. When dysphasia is severe, speech therapy is rarely helpful.

Brain tissue, once destroyed, does not heal. In the area of stroke, therefore, prevention is crucial. Fortunately, there are several things that you can do:

1.  Make sure, if you have high blood pressure, to get it treated (see chapter 5).

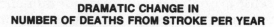

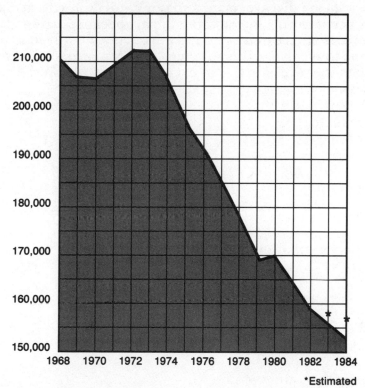

Source: National Center for Health Statistics

2. Take preventive measures against atherosclerosis (see chapter 8).
3. Be alert to warnings of stroke.
4. Do not smoke.

## DECLINE IN INCIDENCE OF STROKES

The stroke rate has fallen for several reasons. First, hypertension is a major contributing factor to stroke, and effective therapy for high blood pressure clearly reduces the likelihood of a stroke. Second, modification of lifestyle to prevent athero-sclerotic disease probably has had a major influence on stroke. Atherosclerosis is an important contributor to stroke. Third, rheumatic heart disease, once a major contributor to stroke, has now become very uncommon, in part because streptococcal infections are treated early and effectively. Finally, doctors have come to recognize the warning signs of a stroke and have treatments that are effective in preventing a stroke in the person at risk.

# 15

## Peripheral Arterial Disease

For reasons that are not clear, atherosclerotic disease involves the lower aorta and the arteries to the legs much more often than the upper aorta and the arteries to the arms. Although a sudden blockage of an artery to an arm or a leg can occur, typically due to an embolism (a clot traveling through the bloodstream from some other place in the body), slowly progressive blockage (occlusion) is much more common.

### SYMPTOMS

The most common symptoms of peripheral arterial disease occur during exercise and are termed "intermittent claudication" (that is, pain that occurs in muscular groups that have an inadequate blood supply, when the need for a blood supply is increased by exercise). The discomfort is often experienced as a cramp that occurs with activity and disappears within one or two minutes after stopping the activity. Weakness may also be noted. The cycle of walking, pain, and rest tends to be relatively constant. Many people note that the problem is more severe in the morning; the reasons are not clear.

The muscle groups involved, and the associated symptoms, reflect the level at which the blood vessel blockage has occurred. (Typical locations for blockage are shown in figure 26.) For example, when the pain during exercise involves the hip, the thigh, and the buttock and is associated with impotence, it suggests that the lower aorta has been occluded. With occlusion further along in the arterial tree, the pain may be restricted to the thigh and calf or the calf itself.

With more severe occlusion or occlusion at multiple levels,

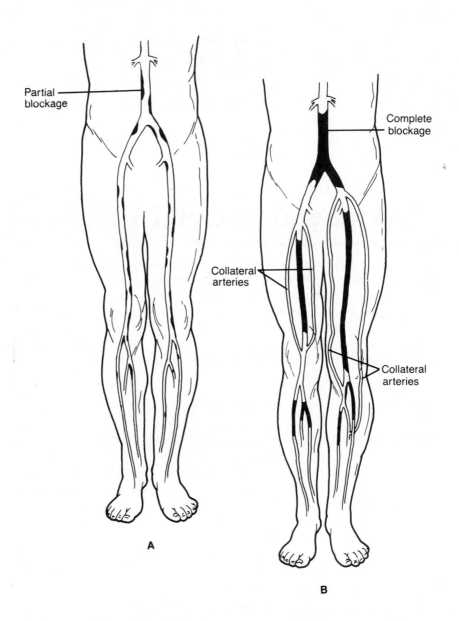

Partial
blockage

Complete
blockage

Collateral
arteries

Collateral
arteries

A

B

**Figure 26.   Peripheral Vascular Disease**

When a complete blockage occurs **(B)**, the nutrition of the lower limb is maintained
by collateral arteries, which are a kind of detour available for blood around the
blocked area. The availability of the collateral arteries determines the adequacy of
nutrition beyond the area of blockage.

peculiar feelings in the skin, numbness, or continuous pain in the toes or foot may occur. Ulceration of the skin and gangrene of the toes and foot are common when the disease reaches an advanced stage. Fortunately, once again, much can be done to prevent or delay that stage.

When an individual has diabetes mellitus, peripheral arterial disease is common. Its symptoms are different, in that the diabetes mellitus influences the nerves to the limb, so there may be a loss of pain sensation. The result is often a painless ulceration.

Color and temperature changes also occur in the limb with an occlusion. If it is a sudden occlusion, the limb is typically white and cold. With more gradual blockage, there are changes in the hair and nails that reflect a poor blood supply, and the limb is often very red when it is allowed to hang over the edge of the bed.

## MEDICAL MANAGEMENT

Evaluation includes measurement of blood pressure at multiple points along the limb. Arteriography is also used, as for coronary artery disease and cerebral vascular disease.

Many individuals can remain stable with medical therapy, adjusting their lives appropriately and avoiding the need for reconstructive arterial surgery. Indeed, surgery is usually limited to those who suffer a substantial limitation in walking, sufficient to affect their livelihood or leisure activities. As in the case of angina pectoris (see chapter 9), transluminal angioplasty—opening the vessel through inflation of a balloon on a specially prepared catheter—has been widely used, with very real success. In general, the results have compared favorably with the results of surgery, though since the procedure is newer, the follow-up information is of shorter duration than for surgery.

### Reversing the Risk Factors

As in every other form of atherosclerotic disease, reversal of risk factors is important. Perhaps the most important is stopping smoking.

Exercise training probably produces the most clear benefit in terms of increased exercise tolerance for individuals with intermittent claudication—once they deal with the fear that ex-

---

**REVERSING RISK FACTORS FOR
PERIPHERAL ARTERIAL DISEASE**

1. Quit smoking.
2. Join an organized exercise training group.
3. Make sure to follow up on the exercise program by assessing your progress every four to six months.

---

ercise will bring on the leg pain associated with walking.

A group training class can break this cycle, providing both a morale booster and help with an organized recovery program. The training program generally means attending a physiotherapy clinic once a week for at least four weeks. The sequence typically involves exercise at a level of manageable intensity, with appropriate rest periods. Supervised exercises are designed to increase power and mobility of the legs.

Follow-up is important. Most often, people are invited to return to the exercise program at intervals of four to six months to assess how much improvement has occurred. Deterioration or lack of improvement is often an indication for angioplasty or surgery.

## Drug Treatment

Drugs of various sorts have been tried for peripheral arterial disease for many years. Vasodilators, such as those prescribed for high blood pressure (see chapter 5), have been disappointing. Indeed, some drugs used for high blood pressure treatment, especially the vasodilators and beta-blockers, tend to reduce blood flow to the limbs and may make claudication worse.

Perhaps the most promising solution has been the introduction of a new drug, pentoxifylline. This is the first drug approved by the FDA in the United States for the treatment of peripheral arterial disease. It decreases blood viscosity (making the blood less thick and sticky) and may inhibit the clotting action of platelets. In carefully controlled studies, it had a measurable impact on the distance people could walk. It is best used in conjunction with a program that includes exercise and a reduction of risk factors. A research drug, kentanserin, is also showing promise in the treatment of peripheral arterial disease in some patients.

Although surgery and angioplasty have come a long way, prevention is still the most important aspect of peripheral arterial disease, as is the case in heart attacks and strokes.

# 16

## Varicose Veins and Phlebitis

Two conditions related to the circulatory system involve the legs primarily, though other parts of the body can be affected. These diseases are varicose veins and phlebitis.

### VARICOSE VEINS

Although varicose veins (prominent, distended veins easily visible under the skin) are common, especially in women, they are not life-threatening. For most people, the primary problem with these veins is cosmetic. For others, there may be aching in the legs and local edema (swelling), especially after prolonged standing or exercise. The edema usually subsides overnight.

The veins have valves that open to allow blood to flow to the heart and close to prevent the blood from traveling backward. If a valve between the surface and deep leg veins fails, blood flows backward into the surface vein, and the vein swells and becomes varicose. The valve can become damaged from a clot. (See figure 27.) The failure of these valves can lead to sustained edema, brownish discoloration of the skin, and fibrosis (hardening of the skin due to formation of fibrous tissue).

#### Treatment of Varicose Veins

Simple measures are usually sufficient to treat most varicose veins. They include frequent periods of rest while keeping the limbs elevated and external pressure provided by elastic stockings or bandages. Obstruction of the veins by tight garments such as a girdle or garters should be avoided.

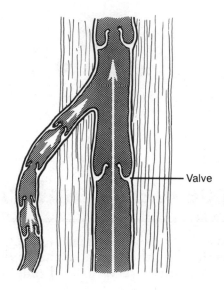

Valve

**Figure 27.   Normal Blood Flow in Veins**
Blood flow goes forward, and competent valves prevent a backward flow of blood.

In more severe or advanced cases, surgery is involved. The veins can be cut and tied off to stop the backward flow of blood and thus relieve swelling (see figure 28). Alternatively, an injection can be used to close off the swollen veins (see figure 29). The clot formed by the injection takes on some of the failed valve's job—closing off blood flow and reducing swelling. This approach is simple, inexpensive, and effective.

When ulcers are present as a complication of long-standing incompetent veins, it may be necessary to remove that portion of the skin and carry out skin grafting to eliminate the ulceration.

## THROMBOPHLEBITIS

Thrombophlebitis (commonly known as phlebitis) is a condition in which blood clots form from stagnant blood in varicose surface veins, typically those of the leg, and is often accompa-

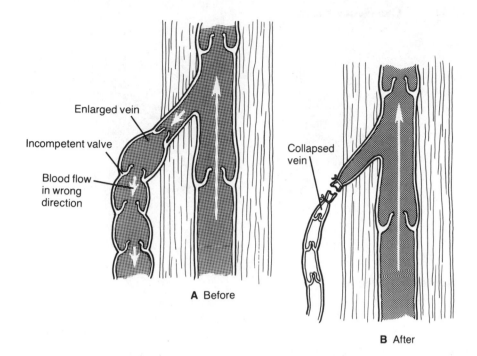

**A** Before

**B** After

**Figure 28.   Effect of Tie-Off Operation on Varicose Veins**

Because of incompetent valves, the blood flow and the pressure delivery in the varicose vein **(A)** is in the wrong direction, and the result is a progressive enlargement of the vein. The effect of the tie-off operation is shown, with resulting collapse of the varicose vein **(B)**.

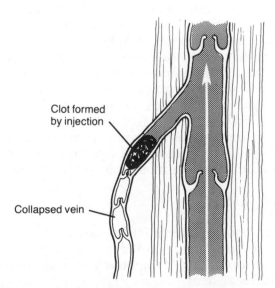

**Figure 29.   Effect of Injection Treatment on Varicose Vein**

An injection has been made to close the varicose vein through clotting.

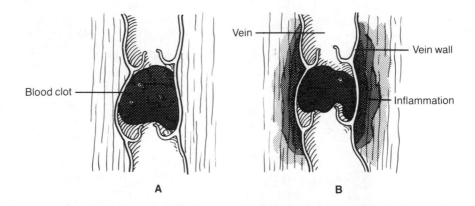

**Figure 30.   Phlebitis**
Phlebitis occurs when blood clots in the vein, and the wall of the vein becomes inflamed. The result is local tenderness, swelling, heat, and pain.

nied by inflammation of the venous wall (see figure 30). It is common, especially in women, and becomes more common with increasing age. Bed rest makes thrombophlebitis more likely, as does pregnancy.

Many people with phlebitis are unaware that they have the condition. The first indication may be chest pain and coughing of blood because a blood clot from the leg veins has floated to the lung (pulmonary embolism). When symptoms are present, typically there is pain in the region of the veins that contain blood clots and are inflamed and swelling below the level of the obstruction. When thrombosis occurs high in the leg, the entire limb typically becomes swollen and the other veins in the leg distended.

Because thrombophlebitis often has no local symptoms, X-ray diagnosis through injection of dye into the venous system may be required. Other tests are available to identify clots.

## Treatment of Phlebitis

When phlebitis is superficial, involving the veins under the skin, local measures usually suffice, including the administration of anti-inflammatory drugs such as indomethacin along with rest and local heat.

When the deep veins are involved, anticoagulants (agents

that prevent or reverse blood clots) are widely used. The reason is the risk of pulmonary embolism, which is the movement of a blood clot to the lung. Elevation of the limb and local heat are also prescribed.

Typically, bed rest is continued until local signs of inflammation, especially tenderness and swelling, subside. Generally, after a week or two, the person is allowed to walk but advised to wear elastic stockings. Resumption of ordinary activity typically follows by a week or two. Anticoagulant drugs are generally prescribed for two to three months.

Many physicians recommend the use of one of the new agents that break up blood clots in the treatment of thrombophlebitis. That use, for several days, is still controversial, however. One by-product of phlebitis is varicose veins, caused by the deep vein damage (see figure 31).

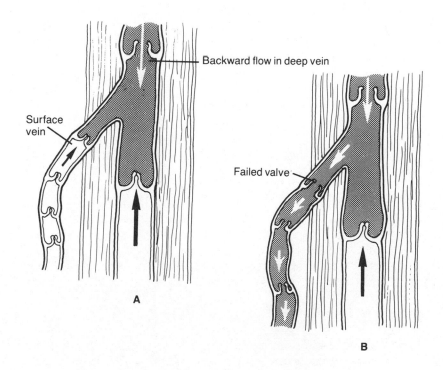

Backward flow in deep vein

Surface vein

Failed valve

A

B

**Figure 31.  Varicose Vein Caused by Deep Vein Damage**
Backward flow in a deep vein caused by a clot can lead to a varicose vein.

As in every other aspect of medicine, prevention is better than treatment. Early exercise following surgery—once considered heresy and now widely encouraged—reflects the attempt to reduce the likelihood that a blood clot to the lung will occur. There is every reason to believe that the program has been very successful.

# 17

## Conditions That Influence Treatment of Cardiovascular Disease

The body is an integrated system, and problems involving the heart or the circulatory system do not always exist in isolation. Indeed, it is not uncommon for people over the age of fifty to be receiving care for more than one chronic condition. Although there is almost an infinite number of combinations of conditions, the more common the conditions are, the greater the likelihood they will occur together. The National Center for Health Statistics keeps track of the frequency of medical problems and recently published information on the ten most frequent chronic conditions in middle-aged individuals and in the elderly (see the chart on page 225).

Hypertension, heart conditions, varicose veins, and arteriosclerosis represent four of the top ten categories.

### ARTHRITIS

The most common problem was arthritis, which was present in 495.8 per thousand persons, or a frequency of just under 50 percent. How might arthritis influence the treatment of diseases of the heart and circulatory system? The most common form of arthritis for older people, osteoarthritis involving the hips and knees, can have a profound influence on physical activity. Substantial emphasis has been given in this book to the importance of regular exercise, with a brisk walk selected as the best example. It makes little sense, obviously, to recommend a brisk daily walk to a person whose knees or hips preclude that activity. The best choice is an alternative, such as swimming.

223

### Drugs Used for Arthritis and Cardiovascular Disease

Drugs widely used for arthritis are also important for the circulation. Nonsteroidal anti-inflammatory agents (aspirinlike drugs) are widely used in the treatment of arthritis and can provide substantial relief. These drugs limit the ability of the kidney to handle sodium and water, so the body retains more salt. For the person with some heart failure or some hypertension that has been nicely controlled, the use of a nonsteroidal anti-inflammatory agent such as indomethacin can result in sufficient retention of sodium and water to substantially worsen the cardiovascular condition.

Drug interactions are also important. Virtually every drug employed for the treatment of hypertension, for example, has its action limited when nonsteroidal anti-inflammatory agents are added. The use of a diuretic is almost always required when these agents are prescribed.

The recent introduction of over-the-counter ibuprofen (brand names Nuprin and Advil)—a low-dosage form of a widely used nonsteroidal anti-inflammatory agent—has increased the use of nonsteroidal anti-inflammatory agents substantially and has complicated the treatment of cardiovascular illness.

One solution involves a return to aspirin or buffered aspirin as an analgesic. Although, when used in high doses, buffered aspirin can have the same influence as the more potent, more recently developed drugs, it is possible to adjust aspirin dose more finely. Lower doses of aspirin will often suffice.

## HIGH BLOOD PRESSURE

Nonsteroidal anti-inflammatory agents interfere consistently with the ability of drugs employed for treatment of hypertension to restore a normal blood pressure. There are important implications for treatment of the individual when the hypertension is associated with a heart condition, sinusitis, or diabetes mellitus.

Beta-adrenergic blocking agents can have different effects on different heart conditions. Heart failure may become worse when a beta-blocker is used for the treatment of high blood pressure. Conversely, if the heart condition is angina pectoris, the use of a beta-blocker provides a kind of "two for one" advantage, since both conditions respond favorably to a beta-adrenergic blocking agent.

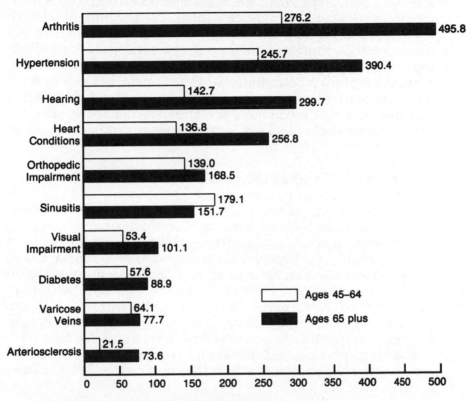

TOP TEN CHRONIC CONDITIONS FOR OLDER PERSONS—
RATES PER 1,000 PERSONS, 1982

Arthritis — 276.2 / 495.8

Hypertension — 245.7 / 390.4

Hearing — 142.7 / 299.7

Heart Conditions — 136.8 / 256.8

Orthopedic Impairment — 139.0 / 168.5

Sinusitis — 179.1 / 151.7

Visual Impairment — 53.4 / 101.1

Diabetes — 57.6 / 88.9

Varicose Veins — 64.1 / 77.7

Arteriosclerosis — 21.5 / 73.6

☐ Ages 45–64
■ Ages 65 plus

Source: National Center for Health Statistics, 1982 HIS Survey.

## SINUSITIS

Sinusitis is an associated condition to watch because many of the medicines employed for the treatment of sinusitis tend to raise blood pressure and hence can make hypertension worse or interfere with the action of antihypertensive drugs.

## DIABETES MELLITUS

In the same way, the presence of diabetes mellitus with hypertension—a frequent pair of coexisting conditions—can influence the choice of treatment. Thiazide diuretics tend to raise blood sugar and can aggravate the diabetes mellitus condition. Beta-blockers, though effective, can mask the signs of too low a blood sugar, a drawback for a diabetic on insulin who is overtreated with insulin or misses a meal. For the individual with diabetes mellitus who also has peripheral arterial disease, another common combination, the use of a beta-adrenergic blocking agent, because of a reduction in blood flow to the limbs, makes leg pain substantially worse. For an individual with hypercholesterolemia, struggling to lower blood cholesterol through diet and medicines, the cholesterol-raising effect of thiazides and beta-blockers is obviously a problem.

## CHRONIC LUNG DISEASE

Also a common problem in the United States is chronic lung disease, whether it be asthma or chronic destructive pulmonary disease related to cigarette smoking. Should it exist with angina pectoris, the bronchodilators used to open the narrowed bronchial tree to ease breathing can have a bad influence on the heart. Conversely, the use of beta-blockers to control angina pectoris or hypertension can make asthma or bronchospasm more severe. If an individual is short of breath because of lung disease and also develops congestive heart failure, which also causes shortness of breath, breathlessness becomes more of a problem early in the course of the heart failure.

---

**BETA-ADRENERGIC BLOCKING AGENTS**

Good for
- high blood pressure
- angina pectoris

Bad for
- heart failure
- diabetes mellitus
- high blood cholesterol
- chronic lung disease

## HYPOTHYROIDISM

An underactive thyroid, hypothyroidism, is also increasingly common with increasing age. Treatment of hypothyroidism with thyroid replacement can precipitate angina pectoris for someone with coronary artery disease, as the metabolic demands of the heart are increased by the thyroid replacement.

## KEEPING INTERACTIONS IN MIND

A number of other problems are less obvious. The individual who has arthritis involving his or her hands may have very real difficulty in opening certain screw-top pill bottles, making it harder to follow a treatment plan faithfully.

What can a person do about all these interactions? One useful action is to draw the attention of your physician and pharmacist to the presence of associated illnesses. It is a very good idea to have all your medications with you whenever you visit your doctor. It is an equally good idea to have all your prescriptions at one pharmacy and to keep a list of the prescriptions so that the pharmacist can review them. This is especially important when a prescription for a new drug is written. No physician, and no pharmacist, minds being asked whether the drugs have any interactions.

This has been a limited examination of a very large number of possible combinations of illnesses and medications. There are many more, less common, interactions. The important thing is to insure that the implications of their joint presence are not forgotten when treatment plans are being devised—especially when you are seeing more than one doctor.

# 18

On Changing Lifestyle

Perhaps the greatest contribution to health made by the popular press has involved informing the public about the contribution of bad habits to disease and death. Although there are frequent reports on "breakthroughs" and true breakthroughs are rare, and too often the wheat and the chaff are separated poorly, the popular press has had a measurable impact on public education. Over the past fifteen years, for example, there has been a progressive fall in the consumption of food that contains a great deal of cholesterol—why else would the price of eggs and beef, as an example, have changed so little over the past decade when the cost of so many items has risen?

The impact of information on public health is measurable. A major trial called "MrFit," the multiple risk factor intervention study, was designed to measure how much effect reducing smoking, lowered cholesterol level, and lowered blood pressure would have on heart attack and death rate. Those individuals who were enrolled as a control group, but not given a special program, showed a progressive decline in blood pressure, body weight, serum cholesterol, and cigarette use. No one doubts that this reflected the impact of public education and the public's response.

But it is also true that many reading this book continue to have a problem with overweight; a sedentary life; the use of cigarettes; the abuse of alcohol; and an excessive intake of saturated fats, cholesterol, and salt—an unhealthy lifestyle. One can be confident, furthermore, that virtually everyone who is overweight, for example, has tried multiple times to lose weight. Indeed, the common story involves periodic dramatic weight loss followed by an interval of equally dramatic weight gain.

To complicate matters, these problems often occur in

According to the National Centers for Disease Control:
- 10 percent of Americans have *uncontrolled* high blood pressure.
- 18 percent smoke a pack of cigarettes every day.
- 59 percent exercise less than three times a week, for twenty minutes per session.

Lack of exercise may be a particularly troublesome risk factor for heart disease, researchers at the NCDC note, because it is so widespread.

clusters. The sedentary individual, for example, is often the same individual who is overweight, smokes, uses alcohol to excess, and ignores what he or she already knows about a judicious diet.

What can be done about it? Although no one would say that changing behavior is easy, it is possible.

## RECOGNIZE THE PROBLEM

The first step, of course, is to recognize the problem and, with that awareness, accept the fact that it is worthwhile to change your behavior. Being aware includes coming to grips with the fact that changing behavior is a skill—a skill that can be learned. Learning involves practice.

## FIND NEW WAYS TO RESPOND TO CUES

Behavior is a chain of events, starting with some cue, or signal, that prompts a certain kind of behavior. These cues are often social and environmental, and the important next step is to identify clearly what these cues are. It may be helpful, and often is, to establish a list of these cues and build on the list.

Learning to avoid or modify the situation that provides the cues can be very helpful. As one example, if certain social situations lead to cigarette smoking, or to injudicious intake of alcohol along with other items high in calories, they can be avoided or alternative behavior invented. The widespread popularity of certain bottled waters, taken as a kind of cocktail with ice and a twist of lime, provides an excellent example. There is something festive about ordering such a drink, and one does not stand out in company with a cocktaillike glass in hand, and yet a substantial number of calories are avoided, as well as another alcoholic drink.

The use of carrot sticks in place of cigarettes or candy is another well-known substitution.

## ESTABLISH BOTH SHORT-TERM AND LONG-TERM GOALS

The next step involves establishing a series of goals, short-term and long-term, and a series of target dates for achieving those goals. Taking losing weight as an example, it is important that the short-term goals be the change in *behavior* and *not* specifically the change in weight. It is equally important to take the long view in establishing goals.

Take another example. An individual who stands 5 feet 4 inches tall, and weighed 125 pounds on graduation from high school some thirty years ago, might weigh 185 pounds today. Those sixty pounds were gained over about thirty years, very *gradually* and with a series of ups and downs.

Let us say that the decision to lose weight was prompted by embarrassment about wearing a bathing suit at the beach. The long-term goal might be to lose half of those sixty excess pounds by late next spring; a weight loss of thirty pounds in ten months involves the loss of three pounds a month, a not-too-difficult series of short-term goals.

The short-term goal would be to establish a change in behavior that would permit achieving the long-term goal. In the case of weight loss, there are several steps. The first involves carefully identifying those factors that contributed to the difficulty in losing weight. For many people, one problem is a sedentary life. The short-term goal would be to establish a daily

---

According to the recent survey done by the Wheat Industry Council, Americans are, in total, 2.3 billion pounds overweight. At any given moment, approximately 28 percent of all Americans are on a diet.

Weight loss is not a problem that anyone is alone with.

pattern of physical activity that would permit the burning of 200–300 additional calories. A three-mile walk, or three one-mile walks, burns 300 calories. At a brisk pace, that can be performed in well under one hour. (The details of walking as exercise are described in chapter 8.)

Example: <u>Losing a Pound—One Day at a Time</u>

To lose a pound in weight, you have to burn 3,500 calories more than you have consumed. To lose a pound each week, then, you must burn 500 calories a day more than you have eaten. The exercise program that was the first step in changing behavior already took care of half those calories. How do you find the other half? Complicated diets really are not necessary. Virtually everyone knows his or her problem area.

For some, it is 600 calories in alcohol, often taken early in the evening. For others, it is a rich snack food taken during the day as "quick energy," or a junk food lunch of hamburger, fries, and a thick shake (two out of every five dollars spent on eating out goes for fast food). For some, it is the breakfast of bacon and eggs with home fries and buttered toast eaten in a diner. For many, it is the rich desserts at lunch and dinner or the tendency to continue snacking through the evening. A rigorous diet is not required to deal with a calorie problem, nor is an upheaval in your life.

---

### CALORIE EXPENDITURES OF VARIOUS ACTIVITIES

| Activity | Calorie Cost per Hour |
|---|---|
| Archery | 168 |
| Bowling | 190 |
| Calisthenics | 330 |
| Cycling | 401 |
| Golf | 223 |
| Jogging | 700 |
| Swimming | 530 |
| Volleyball | 210 |
| Walking | 334 |

---

**LOSING WEIGHT—THE ODDS GET BETTER**

Dr. George L. Blackburn, chief of the Nutrition/Metabolism Laboratory at Harvard Medical School, says, "People who keep their weight off for two years do better at keeping it off for five years, and the odds keep getting better. . . . Hunger usually drops in the second year."

If you can identify the most comfortable place to find those 200–300 calories each day, the rest of the day is left essentially unchanged. You need not be hungry, irritable, lacking in energy, or inefficient. If breakfast was the problem, the unacceptable can be replaced with a bowl of oatmeal and fruit, or fruit and bran muffins, or some sensible alternative. If the problem was a junk food lunch, that can be replaced by a thirty- to forty-five–minute brisk walk and a more sensible lunch that includes tuna salad, vegetables and fruit, and skim milk. Where you find the calories really does not matter (as long as you don't cut the essential nutrients out of your diet); what matters is that you establish a new pattern. The 500 calories are found in a combination of exercise and recognizing the problem source of "junk" calories.

Obviously, if you are to lose weight very gradually, as this program recommends, you cannot make your short-term goals frequent measurements of weight on the scale. The short-term goal clearly has to be the change in behavior itself.

## KEEP TRACK OF CHANGES IN BEHAVIOR

One useful device for monitoring your behavior involves establishing a journal—a diary of events, thoughts, and feelings.

You can begin the journal with a description of your overall objective, long-term goals and short-term goals. You can provide feedback for yourself in the journal through regular self-monitoring. Indeed, it has been suggested that the more novel the feedback system, the more interesting for the individual using it. Charts, graphs, and marks on the calendar are devices that have been used successfully.

### · JOURNAL ·

*January 4: Well, I have finally done it. All my clothes were tight before Thanksgiving, and I seem to lose all restraint during the holidays. I ate too much and too often. I drank too much and too often, and I sat around whenever possible. On New Year's Day, I weighed 186 pounds, about 7 pounds more than I weighed in mid-November, and every item of clothing was tight. This time, my resolution was going to happen.*

*Dr. Smith suggested that I break the habit of crash diets and develop long-term goals. The long-term goal that we agreed on was the loss of about 25 pounds by my summer vacation next July so that I can have new outfits—and be less disgraceful in a bathing suit (we didn't discuss that).*

*The short-term goal was a change of behavior. I am to walk, briskly, at least three miles every day. We decided together that I was sufficiently fit to begin with that, and that I should strive to cover the three to four miles in an hour—though he didn't think it likely that I could do that at the beginning. The second short-term goal was to remove about 300 calories a day from my diet. That could be achieved, in my case, by replacing the cocktail that I have when I get home from work with some seltzer and a twist of lemon, and by having fruit as my dessert at lunch or dinner. Breakfast and lunch seem to be fine.*

*If I can burn 200 to 300 extra calories every day, and reduce my intake by 200 to 300 calories every day, I should lose about a pound a week. He cautioned that I not focus on the scale because the short-term goals were not a visible weight loss evident in a day but rather a change in behavior. He assured me that the weight loss would follow, along with feeling more fit.*

*This journal is his suggestion. I am to use it often enough that I can keep track of how I am doing, and use it to help me correct when I slip.*

He told me that everyone slips occasionally and that the important thing was to get back on track as quickly as possible. He suggested that I keep a graph of my weight at about weekly intervals, and that I indicate on that graph how many days of the week I manage to get my walk in.

*This time, I am going to do it.*

*January 8:* I have managed to walk every day, even though the weather has been cold. When it was really cold on Saturday, I took my walk at the Chestnut Hill Mall. The walk is fun, but I miss having a drink when I get home and slipped rather badly at that party Saturday night. On the other hand, I was very good Sunday. I haven't weighed myself yet and have decided to wait until next Saturday.

*January 21:* I slipped rather badly the last two days. Cocktails and dessert at a business lunch, cocktails in the evening, a disastrously rich dessert at the end of dinner—and I haven't walked for two days. I was doing so well, I will not lose this time. Tomorrow I will walk twice and will have a fruit salad for both lunch and dinner.

*January 25:* I had a great weekend. The weather was mild, and I decided that I wanted to take a two-hour walk, and so I did—all the way into town. I treated myself to a pot of hot tea and a bran muffin and walked all the way home. Who could have imagined that I would be doing that in less than four weeks! I have lost 6 pounds, which is rather more weight loss than I expected, but Dr. Smith told me that the weight I just put on might come off a little more easily, and not to focus on the weight too much. My clothes certainly feel better.

*March 26:* I have had a bad four days. The pressure of getting everything ready for the tax accountant has had me eating poorly, and I have done no walking at all. It has been weeks since I slipped for more than a day, and I will not let this slide. The weather has turned beautiful, and I am going to take a long walk on the Charles River today and tomorrow. I am also going to eat small portions of everything other than vegetables for the next three days until I have "earned" my next meal. I have lost 15 pounds, and I haven't felt this good, or felt this good about me, in years. This time I am in it for the long term.

*March 28:* I have had three marvelous days. Funny, but I think I actually get more work done when I program some time for the brisk walk, and I certainly get more done in the afternoon when I take a walk at lunchtime and finish at a salad bar. I do have to stop talking about all of this, though, because I fear that I am becoming a bore. Even those who love me, and are thrilled that I am so happy, clearly want to change the subject when I start! I am not really gloating—it is just that I want everyone that I love to feel as good as I do!

*April 11:* I haven't written in my journal because I have felt little need to. I have had no slips and find myself walking my three miles very much more quickly than I used to, and more easily. In fact, I am becoming a little concerned that it may not be enough cardiovascular fitness! I will have to remember to ask Dr. Smith how to tell when my exercise is aerobic. I haven't weighed myself for a couple of weeks, but my clothes are definitely becoming a little baggy. In fact, I put on a pair of slacks on the weekend that I hadn't been able to wear for a long time. I don't think I will weigh myself for a couple of weeks because I want to enjoy a large change. And I do have to think about what kind of bathing suit I want to buy for this summer.

## COPE WITH RELAPSE

The journal also provides a way of dealing with relapse. Of course, most people will give in to temptation on occasion and feel guilty. The journal provides a means of identifying relapse and reduces the likelihood that a temporary setback will become a new and negative pattern. If the new pattern has involved a three-mile walk every day, for example, and two or three days of bad weather have broken the pattern, a note in your journal will remind you of that fact and prompt a response. As one example, you can choose to visit a covered mall the next day and resolve to begin your daily walks again. Indeed, a journal can become an important element in the change in behavior; for those who have not kept a journal, doing so is a new behavior.

## REWARD YOURSELF

What about the reward? Too often the reward is distant. A brand-new wardrobe when one has lost sixty pounds is clearly a wonderful reward, but it is a reward that must be waited for. If the change in behavior involves reduced spending on cigarettes, alcoholic beverages, or snack foods, one pleasant reward can involve spending the equivalent amount on some luxury item that you might not otherwise have purchased. With the money your healthy habits save you, you can treat yourself to theater tickets, long-distance telephone calls, or a massage. In a relatively short time, your reward can also be knowing you have met your own goals.

## FIND SUPPORT

Support is important. What can you do in search of support? Alcoholics Anonymous has taught a great deal about the importance of support groups. Joining a group of people who share the same problem can help, especially when relapse occurs. There are a number of organizations that deal with overweight, cigarette smoking, family problems, and drug addiction. They can be located through recommendations from your doctor, chats with friends and relatives, a hospital social service department, ads in the newspaper, or the telephone directory.

## MANAGE STRESS

Stress management is another important aspect of behavioral change. Whether abuse of alcohol, cigarette smoking, or binge eating or other self-destructive eating patterns is the problem, stress often represents an important underlying factor. Awareness must be considered the first step in stress management.

### Become Aware of the Trigger

Again, you begin by identifying the situations that provoke stress. If you are aware of the stress triggers, and anticipate them, the situations may be less stressful.

### Learn to Limit the Reaction to Stress

Often relatively minor events can lead to emotional and physiological responses that are out of proportion to the events themselves; it is your perception of the events that is often important. Awareness—literally talking to yourself about how important or unimportant these events really are—will often make it possible to deal with events more calmly.

Some events, such as the death of a loved one, are worthy of an all-out reaction. But many of the things that provoke stress

---

**RELAXATION RESPONSE**

- Sit in a comfortable position.
- Close your eyes and relax your muscles.
- Focus on your breathing. Breathe slowly and naturally.
- Select a word, prayer, or phrase, such as the number "one" (or, even better, a word or phrase that is rooted in your belief system. . . . Then, repeat it silently or see it in your mind's eye each time you exhale.
- When outside thoughts intrude during the meditation, disregard them by saying, "Oh, well," and return to the word or prayer you've selected. It's essential always to maintain a passive, relaxed style in dealing with any interruptions.

—Dr. Herbert Benson. From *Beyond the Relaxation Response* by Herbert Benson, M.D., with William Proctor, Times Books. New York: The New York Times Book Co., Inc., 1984.

**EXERCISE AND THE HEART**

| Levels of Conditioning | Activity | Cardiovascular Benefits |
|---|---|---|
| 1 | Walking 1–2 mph | Not strenuous enough to promote cardiovascular fitness. |
| | Light housework | Too sporadic and mild to provide adequate dynamic exercise. |
| 2 | Golf, using cart | Improves arm strength, but not vigorous enough to build cardiovascular endurance. |
| | Bowling | Not continuous enough for effective conditioning. |
| | Walking 3 mph | Sufficient for someone with a low exercise capacity. |
| 3 | Mopping, vacuuming, cleaning windows | Good endurance training if continuous for 20–30 minutes. |
| | Walking 3.5 mph | Good conditioning exercise. |
| | Bicycling 8 mph | Promotes cardiovascular strength. |
| 4 | Volleyball, badminton | Good endurance activity when played rigorously. |
| | Walking 4–5 mph | Excellent cardiovascular conditioning activity. |
| | Waterskiing | Dangerous for person with known or hidden heart disease. |
| 5 | Ice- or roller-skating | Excellent when performed continuously. |
| | Bicycling 12 mph | Builds endurance, trains cardiovascular system. |
| | Jogging 5 mph | Excellent conditioner. |
| | Downhill skiing | Not continuous enough to build endurance. |
| 6 | Cross-country skiing | Superb dynamic exercise. |
| | Running 6 or more mph | Promotes cardiovascular strength. |
| | Squash, handball | Dangerous to someone out of condition. Can build endurance in skilled player when continuous for 30 minutes or more. |

**POPULAR SPORTS AMONG AMERICANS OVER 50**

| Activity | Participants |
|----------|-------------|
| General exercise | 14.6 million |
| Swimming | 9.3 million |
| Cycling | 7.4 million |
| Golf | 6.1 million |
| Bowling | 5.2 million |
| Walking | 4.3 million |
| Running | 2.8 million |
| Tennis | 1.3 million |

every day turn out—in a calm, retrospective light—not to have been worth the reaction. Commonly it is not the event that is primarily responsible for upsetting us; we are the ones who upset ourselves. You can exploit the journal, once again, to grade the reality and your reaction. If you grade the seriousness of the event on a scale of one to ten, and grade your reaction on a scale of one to ten, it is easy to see when your response has been disproportionate. When a response is easily recognized as disproportionate under one circumstance, you are likely to remember that fact under the next.

### Manage Time to Cut Down on Stress

Management of time is another critical element in reducing stress. Too often we feel pressure because of failure to set priorities. If an individual learns to identify what is really urgent to accomplish in a certain time, he or she can reduce the stress involved in feeling pressured to meet commitments. Indeed, time management teaches us when to say no.

### Relaxation Techniques

Relaxation techniques involving changes in breathing pattern, biofeedback, or formal meditation are generally not required—though many individuals find satisfaction in their regular use. (Biofeedback is a technique for changing behavior by measuring some physical manifestation, such as brain wave electrical activity, and learning to recognize when a certain state of consciousness results in that brain wave pattern. The "feedback" provided by the recording, with practice, appears to help an individual achieve a certain state.)

## More Formal Coping Techniques

Some health maintenance organizations (HMOs) are providing courses in managing stress, in part because they are finding that it saves them money by cutting down on the incidence of stress-related illnesses.

Rather than focusing strictly on meditation, the class might cover a range of coping techniques. One involves becoming aware of the way we breathe when we are relaxed—deeply, slowly, and smoothly—and comparing it with the shallow, quick, superficial breathing that often aggravates stress. It sounds like a very simple lesson. But learning to breathe under stress is a very effective strategy.

The classes might break up into small groups during each session to discuss stress "triggers" in each person's life. The "support" aspect of changing the way we manage stress, by sharing the stories of our efforts each week, is important. In this way, a class can have an advantage over meditation alone.

For maximum benefit, you must do your homework faithfully, keeping a journal of stress triggers, reactions, and the strategies used to reduce stress. Part of the homework may consist of writing short, encouraging notes to yourself and putting them in conspicuous places. Let people crack jokes—if it works, why not?

The instructor may teach formal relaxation exercises— tensing muscles and relaxing them; breathing in, breathing out. You may learn to practice guided imagery, which consists, basically, of imagining yourself in a situation confronting a stress

---

A study conducted at Pennsylvania State University in 1985 concluded that "worrywarts" would be better off worrying each day, regularly, for half an hour, rather than worrying for briefer intervals throughout the day. It found that approximately 15 percent of us are chronically worried, affected by worry for about eight hours a day.

The study concluded that chronic worriers jump from one worry to another, without giving themselves enough time to think the first worry through. It suggests setting aside time each day to keep a "worry journal."

trigger. Often, in a relaxed state, it is easier for the imagination to tap creative solutions to stressful problems.

Each method of learning to reduce stress has its advantages. If you learn to meditate, whatever the specific technique, you will have a resource that you can use independently whenever you feel the need. The structure of a class, on the other hand, is something that offers the support of other people with the same goal.

There is relaxing potential in a good yoga class, or any class that emphasizes stretching. Any kind of exercise provides a release of tension, and there are some forms of exercise that blend into stress-reduction techniques. To find these classes, look into a center for adult education or a fitness center.

## SET YOURSELF UP FOR SUCCESS

Changing behavior demands some success. The more one has accomplished, the greater the confidence one has of continued success. As in many other areas of life, success breeds success.

---

**IF YOU'RE NOT READY TO QUIT—**
**Tips from the Addiction Research Foundation**

The Addiction Research Foundation has published these rules for those smokers who want to reduce their intake of cigarette smoke:

1. Smoke as few cigarettes as possible no matter what their yield (studies show that people who smoke 40 to 50 cigarettes a day have been able to cut back successfully to 10 per day). Also avoid smoking more than two cigarettes per hour at any time of the day.

2. Smoke the lowest-yield cigarettes that you find acceptable, realizing that it may take weeks to get used to the lower yield. The greater the decrease in yields the better; differences of only 2 milligrams tar and 0.1 milligram nicotine are too small to be important.

3. Do not block vent holes on filters.

4. Take fewer puffs per cigarette.

5. Leave longer butts (the last part of a cigarette delivers the highest yields).

6. Avoid inhaling; if you do inhale, take more shallow puffs.

7. Do not hold the cigarette in your mouth between puffs.

---

**SUPPORT FOR QUITTING SMOKING**

The following organizations can help you quit smoking:

**American Lung Association.** Held once a week for seven weeks. $40 to $75 per person. Success rate of about 32 percent. Clinics focus on positive reinforcement and group interaction. Write to American Lung Association, 1740 Broadway, New York, NY 10019.

**American Cancer Society.** "Fresh Start" program held once a week for four weeks. $25 fee refundable upon completion of program. Success rate of 25 to 30 percent. Write to American Cancer Society, 90 Park Avenue, New York, NY 10016.

**SmokEnders.** Moderated by an ex-smoker and SmokEnder graduate, programs feature a gradual reduction in smoking over first five weeks, followed by four weeks of reinforcement after quit date. $295 per person. Meets weekly. Success rate of over 80 percent. Write to SmokEnders, 18551 Von Karmen Avenue, Irvine, CA 92715.

When several behaviors require changing (as might be true in the case of the sedentary individual who is overweight, smokes, drinks too much, and reacts to situations with a disproportionate amount of stress), it may be impossible to change only one behavior to meet your goal. The excellent example of trying to lose weight when one is sedentary and uses alcohol to excess has been cited many times.

Given the importance of success, it makes excellent sense to begin with that which is most easily changed. For most individuals, committing a specific time of the day to a brisk walk is the easiest change to achieve. When the weather is good, and you can walk in an area that is either lovely or interesting, the experience itself provides a remarkable feeling of well-being. When the weather is bad, a covered shopping mall is a good place for that brisk walk.

Once that pattern of behavioral change is established, especially if at the same time the establishment of a journal has provided positive feedback and an opportunity for exploring other problems, it is time to deal with the next issue. If the problem involves continued eating in the evening, you can shift that walk into the early evening, thus "killing two birds with one stone." The same logic applies to a brisk walk at lunchtime, in place of a visit to a high-calorie, fast-food place. As your fitness improves, the desire for cigarettes is likely to recede. Perhaps more important, establishing success in dealing with one aspect of behavior can help in dealing with other aspects.

## IF YOU THINK IT MIGHT HELP, TRY IT

Anything that might be helpful should be tried. In the case of giving up cigarettes, some persons have found that one or two sessions with a hypnotist has been helpful. Others have found that the use of a nicotine gum helps during the crucial early days. For those with a weight problem, the use of low-calorie, non-sugar-containing custards and puddings to replace their standard dessert can be very helpful. Adding a little wine to seltzer—to make a wine cooler, or spritzer—allows one to enjoy the flavor of wine and to participate in a festive atmosphere without feeling left out.

It is extraordinary what a record of accomplishments can achieve. The awareness that changing behavior is a skill that can be learned, with practice, and that you can deal with relapse effectively provides a very powerful starting point for changing the more difficult behavioral problems. The positive feedback provided by the genuine happiness of loved ones and the encouragement that family and friends provide as you adopt a healthier lifestyle helps sustain momentum.

# 19

## Talking to Your Doctor

Despite an enormous quantity of popular literature on health matters, it is striking how little information is provided to help people communicate with their physicians. No one seems to think that it is important, and yet it is a crucial element in your health care.

The fact that people often come to a physician's office because of well-hidden concerns related to the discovery of a lump somewhere or blood in their urine or because of some equally frightening observation is widely recognized. The person visiting the physician's office will often indicate, however, that he or she came for a checkup, or an unrelated matter, and hope that the physician will stumble onto the matter of concern.

The medical history, the conversation between you and your doctor, is the most important element in uncovering and evaluating problems. What can you do to prepare for a visit with your doctor? The first step is obvious. You need a very clear idea concerning what questions you would really like to have answered. What are your real concerns?

### WRITE QUESTIONS DOWN

It is helpful to write questions down. This achieves several goals. First, and most obvious, you are very unlikely to "forget" (though forgetfulness is virtually never the real reason) to ask a question if it is written down. The discipline of sitting down with a pencil often makes it possible to uncover important questions that you are having trouble dealing with. Finally, and often most important, it is often easier to read a question to your doctor rather than look him or her in the eye and ask it directly.

## SET THE AGENDA

Writing questions down often solves some practical problems. The doctor is generally a busy person operating on a tight schedule and will have made judgments about how to distribute the time available for your visit on the basis of your complaints. Bringing up new issues at the end of the allotted time will often leave both you and the doctor feeling frustrated at having dealt with some of the issues inadequately. If you let the doctor know early that you have a number of questions that you would like to deal with, an agenda of your own, a more judicious and efficient use of that time can be made. If the list is long and requires more time than is available, physicians will often book a special appointment primarily to deal with those issues. Often it is helpful to arrange that visit so that one's spouse is along, especially when family issues or lifestyle changes are an important part of the medical problem.

## MAKE THE MOST OF YOUR EARLY VISITS

When you are taking medication, it is useful to bring all your prescription bottles with you to an appointment. That can cut down on potential errors in the doctor's records. When a prescription for a new medication is being written, it is reasonable to ask whether the new medication will interact with any of the other medications you may be taking.

A detailed history—your occupation, your exposures to illnesses, childhood diseases, diseases in family members, travel, and all the details that can be important in some situations—is often taken during the early visits. When you are seeing a new physician, having this information written out and bringing copies of earlier documents such as hospital records, office records from prior physicians, electrocardiograms, and X rays can be extremely helpful. Some time invested in obtaining those records will make the first visit to a physician's office a much more useful experience. The best way to make sure that the records arrive on time is to carry them to the doctor's office for that visit. For details of your family's history of illness and

---

**PREPARING TO VISIT THE DOCTOR**

1. Ask yourself, "What are my real concerns?"
2. Make a list of questions before the visit.
3. Bring up your "agenda" at the beginning of the visit.
4. Arrive with your medical records, history, and prescription bottles.
5. Remember, *don't hesitate to ask questions!* Your concerns should be aired.

---

childhood illnesses, it is often helpful to speak to family members.

By the same token, it is useful to keep the records at a physician's office updated. If a family member develops a disease that might be relevant, it is worthwhile writing that down so that the information is at hand at the time of your next office visit.

## ASK QUESTIONS

You have every right to ask your doctor about the risks and benefits of some course of action or some procedure such as a diagnostic test, what alternatives are available, and why he or she recommends one course of action rather than another. You also have the right to know whether a course of action is one that is commonly recommended or is a matter of controversy as well as how expensive a procedure or a medication is. These are common concerns and should be aired. With a little practice at writing down your questions, you may find that the questions soon occur spontaneously!

Some people have difficulty in requesting a second opinion when an important course of action, such as an operation, is being discussed. The issue seems to involve embarrassment, a concern that the physician's competence or judgment is being questioned. It is your life and your well-being that is in question, and there is no such thing as a silly question. One useful approach to opening that issue is to ask whether options exist, what they are, and whether some physicians or surgeons might suggest a different course of action. If the answer to the question is yes, you can then, much more easily, ask for a referral to a physician who could offer a second opinion. You might ask, "If you or a member of your family needed this procedure, what doctor would you consider?"

# 20

# A Special Word to Family Members

Illness in a family member clearly has important implications for every member of the family, but especially for the spouse. Everyone has experienced illness in a family member that is short-lived, self-limited, and not a major threat to long-term health. We make short-term adjustments and soon come back to our lifestyle. Eventually, in every family, an illness occurs that is different in nature. The illness might be short-term but a major threat to life during its evolution. Clearly, a heart attack falls into that category. Even more devastating can be the illness that is not short-lived but rather will remain with that individual for the rest of his or her life. What can family members expect from the person who is ill, and what can they do to help the sick person and themselves cope with the new situation?

## UNDERSTANDING THE FEAR OF BECOMING DEPENDENT

Illness represents a threat to the person who is sick, not only in terms of physical well-being but also in terms of status in his or her social group and in the individual's family. In the adult, illness often forces a return to a position of dependency, a change that is usually accompanied by feelings of apprehension, discouragement, anxiety, and even depression.

An individual who has been active, vigorous, and a full and contributing member of the family and of society finds a loss of that status threatening. It is for these reasons that many

**249**

adults in positions of responsibility express greater concern about the economic and social implications of their illness than about the illness itself.

There are a number of what might be considered normal, and certainly common, psychological defenses that a person exercises against illness. Symptoms tend to be minimized, or even go unmentioned, especially when they are the ones causing the most deep concern. If a person has had a tenuous and uncertain level of confidence, any dependency imposed by the illness may come as a welcome relief from adult responsibility. He or she may appear to "enjoy" the illness and even to resent anything that appears to menace that state, which frees the person from responsibilities. If close family members understand the roots of this response, being supportive is much easier. While the individual who is sick requires substantial support, family members have their needs too.

## MAINTAINING COMMUNICATION

Communication is important. Keeping the lines of communication open to the person who is ill is crucial. It is equally important to maintain good lines of communication with the doctor who is taking care of the patient. That is obviously easiest when the responsible physician has been involved with the family for some time. Whether that is the case or not, it is important to use any opportunity to communicate with the doctor effectively.

You can make best use of your time with the doctor if you have thought out carefully what you would like to know before the meeting and have your questions written down (see chapter 19). Often it is necessary to make a separate appointment to discuss your loved one's medical problem with the doctor. If several family members are involved, it is best if such an appointment is made for all, simultaneously. A busy physician finds it difficult to make the time necessary to communicate with many family members independently.

### Questions for the Doctor

There are a number of questions that virtually everyone would like to have answered. What is going to happen? The answer, of course, cannot be specific. At best, what the physician can provide is a range of possible outcomes and, perhaps, a reasonable guess as to the most likely one. No physician likes to raise false hopes, yet no physician feels sufficiently wise and knowledgeable to suggest such a grim prognosis that no hope is possible. Ultimately, it may become apparent to all concerned that no hope is possible. Another important question involves what the options are in selecting a course of treatment. If options are available, and if the procedures proposed carry some risk, the delicate issue of the second opinion is really not so delicate (see chapter 19).

It is also reasonable to ask the physician what one can do or contribute. Sometimes the contribution involves information. Close family members can help the physician and the patient identify what might be important earlier events. When loss of appetite and weight loss actually began is one example. Family members can help obtain information by remembering and providing the names and telephone numbers of physicians who might have been involved earlier or by uncovering evidence of a similar problem in other family members.

## PARTICIPATING IN TREATMENT

Family members can also be helpful in the treatment. Where the treatment involves a change in behavior or a special diet, achieving the goal virtually always involves family members. The best approach is to incorporate these factors into the family's daily life without making too much of them.

Family members have to remember that changing behavior is not easy. Virtually everyone will slip on occasion. Because the individual who is ill often resents being dependent, an aggressive approach on the part of family members to correct-

---

### QUESTIONS FOR THE DOCTOR

- What is going to happen? (the prognosis)
- What are the options in treatment?
- What doctor can you recommend who could offer a second opinion?
- What can I do to contribute to the treatment?

ing that transgression will often lead to anger and withdrawal. It is much better to be understanding and provide a warm and loving support toward return to "good behavior." Participation is important. If the change in behavior involves giving up cigarettes, that is an opportunity for every family member to give up their cigarettes. If a change in diet is involved, often everyone in the family will benefit from sharing at least elements of that diet. If exercise is the issue, why not make those brisk walks discussed in earlier chapters a family event? It is not unusual for a treatment involving anything other than medication to be useful for everyone, not just the individual whose behavior is being addressed directly.

## TAKING MEDICATIONS— REMINDING PAINLESSLY

The taking of medicines is a special case. One reflection of denial is not to take a medicine. Certainly, many people placed on medications do not take all their pills. Asking a person whether he or she has taken a prescribed medicine is not the best approach. One simple solution involves organizing the medicines into a weekly package. Pharmacies have small plastic containers, called pill organizers, divided into seven transparent sections—one section for each day's medication. That obviously makes carrying medications much easier and makes it easier to remember, and tell, whether they have been taken. Equally, it helps family members see whether that day's medication has been taken without upsetting the individual.

## COPING EMOTIONALLY WITH ILLNESS

Family members have to resist the temptation to infantilize the individual who is sick. Being helpful does not mean taking all duties and responsibilities away. Ill persons require encouragement to do as much as they can, both physically and mentally. The more the person who is sick does, the more he or she can do.

Finally, the healthy family members must free themselves of the guilt that inevitably occurs when they lose patience with the sick family member. Some loss of patience, some anger, and some restlessness are inevitable. If one keeps one's lines of communication open with the sick person, these feelings may occur less frequently and may be kept in proportion, but they will occur. Be gentle with yourself and forgive yourself.

## HELPING WITH FINANCIAL CONCERNS

Family members can also help deal with very real concerns about financial matters. Illness often involves not only a substantial expense but also a sharp reduction in income. Reassurance without substance rarely satisfies the person who is ill—or, indeed, the spouse and other family members who often share the financial concern. What is required is a plan. What can be done to supplement the available resources? What can be done to reduce expenses to the level of available resources? Agencies are available to assist in these matters, and it is important to call upon them.

Major hospitals always have a social services department, as do government agencies. Your local Social Security office might be helpful. For many individuals, workmen's compensation insurance could prove beneficial. Many companies offer opportunities to long-term employees to engage in a new line of work that may be appropriate to their new health status. Many insurance policies contain a disability clause that requires exploration.

See Appendix B for a list of available services and their sources.

Whatever the solution, the fact that something is being done and any bit of encouraging news can be enormously reassuring to the sick person—and, indeed, once again, to the spouse. Eventually solutions will be found—they always are. The fact that they are being sought, actively, and that progress is being made can be helpful for all concerned.

# 21

*✦*

# Progress Against
# Cardiovascular Disease

According to the American Heart Association, deaths from cardiovascular disease have been falling since 1972, and substantially. Between 1972 and 1984, cardiovascular disease mortality fell by 32.5 percent, and that has continued in 1985, with the most up-to-date data indicating a 34.6 percent fall (see page 258). The fall in stroke rate was 47.8 percent between 1972 and 1984, and 48.4 percent in 1985. These significant reductions in mortality are far higher than the decrease in mortality due to noncardiovascular diseases.

Why have these rates been falling? Reduced smoking, dietary awareness, weight control, exercise programs, training in cardiopulmonary resuscitation (CPR), along with new and improved cardiovascular drugs, antihypertensive therapy, coronary care units, mobile coronary units, coronary bypass surgery, and angioplasty have all been contributing factors. Most of these factors include something that *you* can do to prevent heart attack and stroke. The factors under your control play an important part in the progress against cardiovascular disease.

The education programs have been working. Information from the U.S. Department of Agriculture has demonstrated a 27 percent reduction in the consumption of animal fat, with a parallel increase in the consumption of vegetable fats and fish over the past several years. There was a 36 percent reduction in the rate of salt sales, from 2¼ to less than 1½ pounds per capita, between 1972 and 1985. The sale of eggs and butter has also decreased. There is a substantial reduction in cigarette use, especially by adult males; but unfortunately a large number of young women are smoking, so the total reduction is less than one might have wished or predicted.

This is all good news and further evidence that we can influence the length and quality of our lives. But, the news is not all good. An estimated 1.5 million Americans will suffer heart attacks this year, one-third of which will prove fatal within the year. About 5 percent of these heart attacks will occur in persons under the age of forty, and 45 percent will occur in persons under the age of sixty-five.

An estimated 2,169,000 cardiovascular operations and corrective procedures will be performed this year, including over 200,000 coronary artery bypass operations. The total cost, including lost productivity, will be over 85 billion dollars in 1988. Stroke will cost Americans an additional 12.8 billion dollars, and one-third of the stroke-disabled individuals will be wage earners from thirty-five to sixty-five years of age.

Taken in all, the evidence indicates that what has been recommended will work *if* it is employed, but there is a long way to go. Each person needs to control the factors that put that individual at risk. You now have the necessary information to do this—use it!

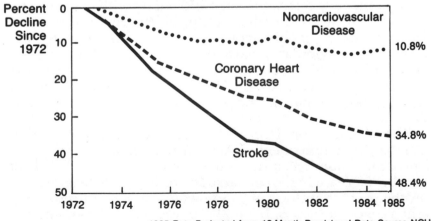

**PERCENT DECLINE IN AGE-ADJUSTED MORTALITY RATES UNITED STATES 1972–1985**

Percent Decline Since 1972

Noncardiovascular Disease — 10.8%

Coronary Heart Disease — 34.8%

Stroke — 48.4%

1972   1974   1976   1978   1980   1982   1984  1985

1985 Rate Projected from 18-Month Provisional Data Source NCHS.

Source: National Center for Health Statistics

**FACTORS IN REDUCTION IN
CARDIOVASCULAR MORTALITY IN THE U.S.**

1. Dietary awareness
2. Exercise programs
3. Weight control
4. Reduced smoking
5. Antihypertensive therapy
6. New and improved cardiovascular drugs
7. Coronary care units
8. Cardiopulmonary resuscitation (CPR) training
9. Coronary bypass surgery
10. Mobile coronary units

# Appendix

# A

## Generic (Chemical) and Brand (Trade) Names of Common Prescription Drugs Used in the Treatment of Cardiovascular Disease

| Generic (Chemical) Name | Brand (Trade) Name |
| --- | --- |
| acebutolol | SECTRAL |
| amiloride | MIDAMOR |
| atenolol | TENORMIN |
| atropine sulfate | ATROPINE-CARE, ATROPISOL |
| bumetanide | BUMEX |
| captopril | CAPOTEN |
| chlorothiazide | DIURIL |
| chlorthalidone | HYGROTON, THALITONE |
| cholestipol | COLESTID |
| cholestyramine | QUESTRAN |
| clonidine hydrochloride | CATAPRES |
| diazoxide | HYPERSTAT IV |
| digitalis | LANOXIN |
| digoxin | LANOXIN, LANOXICAPS |
| diltiazem | CARDIZEM |
| disopyramide phosphate | NORPACE, NORPACE CR |
| enalapril maleate | VASOTEC |
| epinephrine hydrochloride | EPIFRIN |
| ethacrynic acid | EDECRIN |
| furosemide | LASIX |
| gemfibrozil | LOPID |
| guanabenz acetate | WYTENSIN |
| guanethidine | ISMELIN |
| hydralazine | APRESOLINE |
| hydrochlorothiazide | ESIDRIX, HydroDIURIL |
| indomethacin | INDOCIN, INDOCIN SR |
| isosorbide dinitrate | DILATRATE-SR, ISORDIL, SORBITRATE |

| Generic (Chemical) Name | Brand (Trade) Name |
|---|---|
| lisinopril | ZESTRIL |
| lovastatin | MEVACOR |
| methyldopa | ALDOMET |
| metoprolol tartrate | LOPRESSOR |
| minoxidil | LONITEN |
| nadolol | CORGARD |
| niacin | NICOBID |
| nifedipine | PROCARDIA |
| pentaerythritol tetranitrate | PERITRATE |
| pentoxifylline | TRENTAL |
| phenytoin | DILANTIN |
| pindolol | VISKEN |
| prazosin hydrochloride | MINIPRESS |
| procainamide hydrochloride | PROCAN SR, PRONESTYL, PRONESTYL SR |
| propranolol hydrochloride | INDERAL, INDERAL LA |
| qinidine sulfate | QUINIDEX |
| reserpine | SERPASIL |
| spironolactone | ALDACTONE |
| spironolactone and hydrochlorothiazide | ALDACTAZIDE |
| streptokinase | STREPTASE, KABIKINASE |
| terazosin | VASOCARD |
| triamterene | DYRENIUM |
| triamterene and hydrochlorothiazide | DYAZIDE, MAXZIDE |
| trimazosin | CARDOVAR |
| urokinase | ABBOKINASE |
| verapamil | CALAN, CALAN SR, ISOPTIN |

# Appendix

# Home Care Services

Home care allows a sick person to return home from the hospital sooner than might otherwise be possible. Family members are supported in taking care of the sick person. Help is also available for child care and housekeeping, if this becomes difficult for the family.

### WHAT KINDS OF SERVICES ARE AVAILABLE?

**Health Services.** Home care means help with personal care, such as bathing, dressing, dental hygiene, and dressing changes. It provides nutrition services to help address special needs and build proper diets. It offers medical and skilled nursing care, including counseling and administration of prescribed treatments, such as drug therapy or parenteral feeding, lab work, and testing. Home care therapy treatments can include physical therapy to renew or increase movement, occupational therapy to help the patient manage daily tasks at home or work, speech therapy, ostomy therapy, respiratory, IV, or chemotherapy.

**Homemaking Services.** Home care means services to help the individual or family maintain the home. That may mean assisting with meal preparation, housekeeping, laundry, or food shopping. It may mean personal care services. It may involve teaching the family how to budget or to raise a child, or it may mean directly providing child care for an ill parent or the one whose energies are taxed by the care of another ill or disabled family member.

**Social Services.** Home care can help the family cope with problems associated with the care of an ill person and coordinate home care with other community programs affecting the family.

**Hospice Services.** Hospice programs provide physical, social, and emotional care for the terminally ill and their families. They often involve palliative—or pain management—programs to relieve the patient while helping him or her stay alert. Hospice works to maintain the family's quality of life by helping family members keep up as many family activities as practical. It continues to care for the family through the bereavement period.

**Supportive Services.** Home care is much more than health care alone. Some of the important supportive services offered by home care agencies include *adult daily care*, providing supervised activities and meals at specific gathering places; *adult foster care*, which arranges for elderly adults to live with families willing to share their homes; and *adult protective services*, which provide legal and financial counseling to those unable to manage alone.

Home care agencies also offer *respite care*, which arranges for residential care for the ill person for a few hours or a few weeks, giving relief to the family from the pressures of ongoing care. *Pastoral counseling* is another important supportive service, especially for hospice families.

Home care offers *chore services* to help with heavy household tasks. *Home-delivered meal programs* offer nutritious, commercially prepared meals to those who cannot cook for themselves. And *friendly visiting* and *telephone reassurance programs* provide the homebound with the personal contact important in combating loneliness and assuring personal safety.

Agency *transportation and escort programs* offer rides and assistance to elderly or handicapped people who could not otherwise get out into the community.

Increasingly, home care agencies are providing *equipment services*. They will either rent or sell equipment such as walkers, hospital beds, wheelchairs, and oxygen tanks. Some agencies will lend items at little or no cost or arrange for them through community loan closets for those who cannot pay.

## HOW TO CHOOSE A HOME CARE AGENCY

Finding the best home care agency for your needs requires research, but it is time well spent. Quality of care and caliber of personnel will be overriding factors, of course. Fortunately, in most communities families have a wide choice of agencies from which to choose. Some offer sliding-scale fee schedules. Some will accept indigent patients.

Here are some questions to consider when making a decision on what home care agency is best for you:

1. How long has the agency been serving the community?

2. Does my physician know the reputation of the agency?

3. Is it certified by Medicare? Even if your care will not be paid for by Medicare, the fact that an agency is Medicare-certified is one measure of quality. It means that the agency has met certain minimum requirements in financial management and patient care.

4. Is the agency licensed? In most states a home care agency must be licensed by the state, usually by the state health department.

5. Does the agency provide written statements describing its services, eligibility requirements, fees, and funding sources? Often an annual report will offer helpful guidance on the agency.

6. How does an agency choose its employees? Does it protect its workers with written personnel policies, benefit packages, and malpractice insurance?

7. Does a nurse or therapist conduct an evaluation of your needs in the home? What is included—consultations with family members? with the patient's physician? with other health professionals?

8. Is the plan of care written out? Does it include the specific duties to be performed, by whom, at what intervals, and for how long? Can you review the plan?

9. Does the plan provide for the family to undertake as much of the care as is deemed practical?

10. What are the financial arrangements? Can you get them in writing, including any minimum hour or day requirements the agency may have and any extra charges to be involved in the care program?

11. Does the professional supervising your home care plan visit your home regularly? Are your questions followed up and resolved?

12. What arrangements are made for emergencies?

13. What arrangements are made to insure patient confidentiality?

14. Will the agency continue service if Medicare or other reimbursement sources are exhausted?

15. Some people feel that accreditation assures quality of service. Accreditation is a voluntary process conducted by nonprofit professional organizations. Visiting nurse associations and other community nursing groups are accredited by the National League for Nursing/American Public Health Association. The Joint Commission on Accreditation of Hospitals accredits hospitals and their affiliate agencies. And the National HomeCaring Council accredits homemaker–home health aide services.

To locate home care agencies in your community, you might start by asking your doctor, or consult with the hospital discharge planner if home care will follow hospitalization. Agencies will be listed in the Yellow Pages under any of several health-related headings. Your county or city will have listings of publicly funded services. If your community has an information and referral service, check with it. Often information and referral services are affiliated with the local United Way (sometimes called United Fund).

Most states have state home care associations that can help you locate a good agency. The National Association for Home Care (NAHC) can help you contact your state association. Their address is 519 C Street, N.E., Stanton Park, Washington, D.C. 20002.

## FINDING FUNDS WHEN YOU NEED THEM

If you are over the age of sixty-five and have resources amounting to less than $3,000 a year, you may qualify for Medicaid, as well as Supplemental Security Income, under Title 16 of the Social Security Act. Under some circumstances, Title 20 of the Social Security Act, or the Older Americans Act, may entitle you to funds for homemaker–home health aide services. Contact your city or county Office on Aging, local welfare office, or local Social Security office for more information.

If your assets are greater than that, and you are retired, you still qualify for Social Security income and Medicare. Call your local Social Security office for more information.

Medicare pays for some home health services. It covers part-time skilled nursing at home, physical therapy and speech therapy at home, and, when needed, occupational therapy, social services, part-time home health aide services, and medical supplies. It will not cover meals delivered to the home or housekeeping.

If you are under the age of sixty-five, you may qualify for Social Security Disability Insurance if your physical condition makes it impossible for you to work. Each application for Social Security Disability Insurance is reviewed and adjudicated locally. If you are found to qualify, you also are entitled to Medicare, after a waiting period of two years.

If you have private health insurance, home care may be covered under a "Miscellaneous" clause. Health Maintenance Organizations (HMOs) sometimes offer coverage of home care; if they are a federally qualified HMO, they are required to do so. Disability insurance and worker's compensation cover funds for home care under certain circumstances.

Home care is often less expensive than hospitalization because you are paying for only those services that your family needs help in providing.

Some home care agencies receive funding from the United Way, or other community organizations, in order to be able to provide care for fees based on a sliding scale, depending on your income.

## FINDING OUT MORE ABOUT HOME CARE

The following are national organizations that will provide information about home care:

National Homecaring Council
235 Park Avenue South
New York, NY 10003
(212) 674-4990

(The council, in conjunction with the Council of Better Business Bureaus, publishes a pamphlet called *All About Home Care: A Consumer's Guide.* It can be obtained for $1.00 from the above address.)

National Association for Home Care
519 C Street, N.E., Stanton Park
Washington, DC 20002

Visiting Nurse Association of America
518 17th Street #388
Denver, CO 80202

(The national office can furnish information about services provided all over the country by local Visiting Nurse Associations.)

For local information and referrals, contact the following:

- hospital home care and social services departments
- the United Way
- the local Visiting Nurse Association
- local Information and Referral Service. (If there is no such listing in the telephone directory, call your operator for assistance.)
- Family service agencies
- Meals on Wheels
- Religiously affiliated organizations

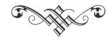

# Index

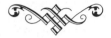

# About the Authors

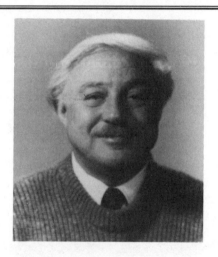

**Norman K. Hollenberg, M.D., Ph.D.,** is Professor and Director of Physiologic Research, Department of Radiology, Harvard Medical School, and Senior Associate in Medicine, Cardiorenal Division, Department of Medicine, Brigham and Women's Hospital. He also serves as consultant to the Children's Hospital Medical Center, Dana-Farber Cancer Institute, Parker Hill Medical Center, New England Deaconess Hospital, and the Veterans' Administration Hospital—all in the Boston metropolitan area.

A physician actively involved in research of treatment for cardio-vascular disease, he has also completed full training in pharmacology and in internal medicine. His responsibility as an associate editor at the *New England Journal of Medicine* in recent years has included the evaluation of important trials of medical therapy.

Dr. Hollenberg is the recipient of numerous scholarships, prizes, medals, and awards and has held memberships in national and international medical societies and organizations. He has edited more than a dozen books, monographs, and journal supplements; served on editorial boards; and written more than 150 original reports and over 100 review articles and book chapters.

He has been a visiting professor in thirty-one countries, with extended stays in Southeast Asia, the Pacific, the Middle East, Africa, and Europe.

Dr. Hollenberg resides with his wife, Deborah, in Brookline, Massachusetts, and has two children—Ilana, with whom he wrote this book, and David.

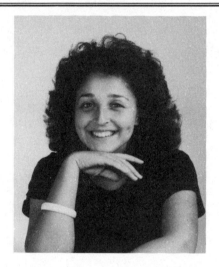

**Ilana B. Hollenberg** graduated summa cum laude from Tufts University and was the recipient of the Departmental Prize in Anthropology. An avid reader and walker, Ms. Hollenberg is the daughter of Norman K. Hollenberg and a collaborator with him on other medical writings. She is currently pursuing a law degree at Stanford University in Stanford, California.

# Other AARP Books

**AARP PHARMACY SERVICE PRESCRIPTION DRUG HANDBOOK**
0-673-24842-9     $13.95 (paperback)
0-673-24887-9     $25.00 (hardcover)

**ALONE—NOT LONELY**
**Independent Living for Women Over Fifty**
by Jane Seskin
0-673-24814-3     $6.95

**CAREGIVING**
**Helping an Aging Loved One**
by Jo Horne
0-673-24822-4     $13.95

**CATARACTS**
by Julius Shulman, M.D.
0-673-24824-0     $7.95

**ESSENTIAL GUIDE TO WILLS, ESTATES, TRUSTS, AND DEATH TAXES, THE**
by Alex J. Soled
0-673-24890-9     $12.95 (paperback)
0-673-24891-7     $19.95 (hardcover)

**FITNESS FOR LIFE**
**Exercises for People Over 50**
by Theodore Berland
0-673-24812-7     $12.95

**GADGET BOOK, THE**
**Ingenious Devices for Easier Living**
edited by Dennis R. La Buda
0-673-24819-4     $10.95

**GOING INTO BUSINESS FOR YOURSELF**
by Ina Lee Selden
0-673-24882-8     $8.95

**HOMESHARING AND OTHER LIFESTYLE OPTIONS**
by Jo Horne with Leo Baldwin
0-673-24886-0     $12.95

**HOW TO PLAN YOUR SUCCESSFUL RETIREMENT**
by AARP Worker Equity Department
0-673-24889-5     $9.95

**INSIDE TRACT, THE**
**Understanding and Preventing Digestive Disorders**
by Myron D. Goldberg, M.D., and Julie Rubin
0-673-24840-2     $9.95

**IT'S YOUR CHOICE**
**Planning a Funeral**
by Thomas C. Nelson
0-673-24804-6     $4.95

**KEEPING OUT OF CRIME'S WAY**
by J. E. Persico with George Sunderland
0-673-24801-1     $6.95

**LIFE AFTER WORK**
**Planning It, Living It, Loving It**
by Allan Fromme, Ph.D.
0-673-24821-6     $6.95

**MEDICAL AND HEALTH GUIDE FOR PEOPLE OVER FIFTY**
by The Dartmouth Institute for Better Health
0-673-24816-X     $14.95

**MYTH OF SENILITY, THE**
by Robin Marantz Henig
0-673-24892-5     $14.95

**NATIONAL CONTINUING CARE DIRECTORY**
**Retirement Communities with Nursing Care**
by American Association of Homes for the Aging
0-673-24885-2     $19.95

**ON THE ROAD IN AN RV**
by Richard Dunlop
0-673-24839-9     $8.95

**OSTEOPOROSIS**
**The Silent Thief**
by William A. Peck, M.D., and
Louis V. Avioli, M.D.
0-673-24837-2    $9.95

**OVER EASY FOOT CARE BOOK, THE**
by Timothy P. Shea, D.P.M., and
Joan K. Smith
0-673-24807-0    $6.95

**PLANNING YOUR RETIREMENT
HOUSING**
by Michael Sumichrast, Ronald G. Shafer,
and Marika Sumichrast
0-673-24810-0    $8.95

**POLICY WISE**
**Insurance Decisions for Older
Consumers**
by Nancy H. Chasen
0-673-24806-2    $5.95

**RETIREMENT EDENS OUTSIDE THE
SUNBELT**
by Peter A. Dickinson
0-673-24836-4    $10.95

**SLEEP BOOK, THE**
by Ernest Hartmann, M.D.
0-673-24825-9    $10.95

**SUNBELT RETIREMENT**
by Peter A. Dickinson
0-673-24832-1    $11.95

**SURVIVAL HANDBOOK FOR WIDOWS**
by Ruth Jean Loewinsohn
0-673-24820-8    $5.95

**THINK OF YOUR FUTURE**
**Retirement Planning Workbook**
by AARP Worker Equity Department
0-673-24893    $24.95

**TRAVEL AND RETIREMENT EDENS
ABROAD**
by Peter A. Dickinson
0-673-24883-6    $16.95

**TRAVEL EASY**
by Rosalind Massow
0-673-24817-8    $8.95

**WALKING FOR THE HEALTH OF IT**
by Jeannie Ralston
0-673-24826-7    $6.95

**WHAT TO DO WITH WHAT YOU'VE GOT**
**Money Management in Retirement**
by Peter Weaver and Annette Buchanan
0-673-24805-4    $7.95

**WOMAN'S GUIDE TO GOOD HEALTH
AFTER 50, A**
by Marie Feltin, M.D.
0-673-24815-1    $12.95

**YOUR VITAL PAPERS LOGBOOK**
by AARP Worker Equity Department
0-673-24833-X    $4.95

For complete information, write
AARP Books, 1900 East Lake Avenue,
Glenview, IL 60025, or contact your
local bookstore.

Prices subject to change.